# Coffee

# Making

# RECIPES

**Brewing Perfection:**
A Comprehensive Guide to
Crafting Irresistible Coffee Creations at Home

## Lucy Abbott

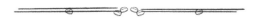
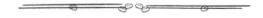

# Table of Contents

vi

# Introduction

Welcome to "Coffee Making Recipes: Brewing Perfection," your go-to resource for learning how to make exceptional coffee at home. A great cup of coffee is more than just a beverage in the busy world we live in daily; it's a ritual, an inspiration, and an opportunity to relish life.

This extensive electronic book is your pass to the world of coffee expertise. Whether you're a seasoned connoisseur or a beginner coffee lover, come along on an extraordinary adventure where we explore the art and science that goes into each brew. We explore the subtleties of coffee beans, explain the tools, and offer detailed instructions to improve your coffee-making process.

You will thoroughly understand the nuances involved in crafting the ideal cup of coffee as you embark on your journey. We consider coffee beans when choosing the best and learning different brewing techniques. Explore the fragrant world of coffee, where each cup reveals a tale of origin, roasting method, and individuality.

This book celebrates the various cultures and customs that have shaped coffee worldwide, not merely a collection of recipes. Explore the vibrant Latin American coffee markets, immerse yourself in Italy's rich espresso culture, and delight in the fragrant delights of Turkish coffee. Explore the relationship between coffee and desserts, master the art of milk foaming, and let your creativity run wild with flavored creations.

This e-book explores the environmental and ethical aspects of coffee manufacturing in addition to pleasing your palate. Find out how making coffee choices can help create a more socially and environmentally conscious world.

"Coffee Making Recipes: Brewing Perfection" is your guide to navigating the fascinating and fragrant world of coffee, whether you're looking for the ideal morning routine or want to wow guests with your barista abilities. A trip where each cup is a masterpiece just waiting to be brewed awaits you, so get ready to go on it.

# Chapter I

## Understanding Coffee Beans

### Types of Coffee Beans

The world of coffee is a fragrant and varied place where different varieties of coffee beans grown worldwide have different flavors and characteristics. Coffee lovers frequently have to sort through the jargon of Arabica, Robusta, and specialty kinds, each providing a different cup experience.

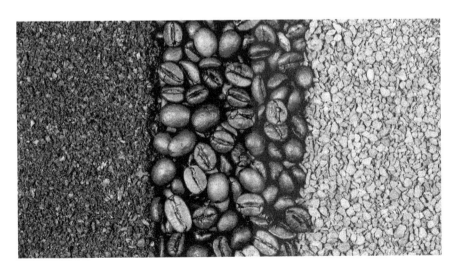

The most well-liked and extensively consumed coffee bean is Arabica, the darling of the coffee world. Arabica beans, prized for their subtle flavors, have a more complex and sweeter flavor profile than Robusta beans. Arabica beans are native to Ethiopia's highlands and grow best in colder climates, where they take longer to mature and develop. The end product is a cup of coffee highly favored by individuals who value a sophisticated and varied taste because it frequently has overtones of flowers, fruits, and wine.

Robusta beans, on the other hand, are distinguished by their solid and assertive qualities. Originating primarily from low-lying areas of Southeast Asia and Africa, robusta beans are hardy plants that tolerate more extreme weather conditions. This toughness results in coffee with more caffeine and a distinctly more robust flavor—occasionally earthy or woody. Beyond its reputation for boldness, robusta is also a key ingredient in espresso blends, adding body and crema to the final product.

Specialty coffee beans are the domain of coffee enthusiasts, going beyond the dichotomy of Arabica and Robusta. These beans are raised above the traditional classifications since they are frequently grown in particular microclimates. Specialty coffee varietals such as Ethiopian Yirgacheffe, Bourbon, and Geisha enthrall coffee enthusiasts with their distinct and sought-after qualities. Geisha is prized for its vivid and flowery notes, which are sometimes compared to those of jasmine or bergamot. It originated in Ethiopia and later flourished in Panama. Conversely, Bourbon had its origins on the island of Bourbon, which is now known as Réunion. It produces a complex cup that strikes a balance between sweetness and acidity.

Ethiopian Yirgacheffe is another exceptional specialty bean that takes you to a coffee's origins. This Yirgacheffe-grown bean reveals a complex dance of floral overtones and citric acidity, making it a favorite among people who value Ethiopian coffee's authentic flavor.

As we travel the world in pursuit of extraordinary coffee experiences, the impact of terroir is apparent. The climate, soil type, and altitude of coffee-growing countries all significantly impact the beans' flavor characteristics. For example, beans from Central America, which are frequently grown at higher altitudes, are prized for their vibrant acidity and subtle fruit overtones. On the other hand, Indonesian beans that grow on volcanic soil have earthy, robust flavors.

Coffee beans come from a world where geography is just one aspect of the story; processing techniques influence the final flavor profile. The process of washing, which entails carefully cleaning and fermenting the beans, brings out their natural qualities. Conversely, the birth or dry method dries the coffee cherries while the beans are still within, adding a fruitier and occasionally wine-like flavor.

In recent years, direct trade and traceability have become more prevalent in the coffee industry. Customers can now follow the path of their "From the farm to the cup: The journey of coffee beans."

thanks to this increased transparency, which strengthens links between coffee consumers and the communities that grow the beans.

In summary, coffee beans are a rich tapestry with many flavors, and each bean has a unique story about how it was grown, harvested, and processed. For those who want more than simply a drink but a sensory experience through the world's most popular morning ritual, the variety of coffee beans, from the high-altitude plantations of Ethiopia to the lush fields of Southeast Asia, offers a limitless exploration. Classic rivals Robusta and Arabica set the tone, but exotic kinds steal the show, beckoning us to taste the subtle nuances that make every cup a memorable experience.

## Coffee Growing Regions

The world of coffee is a rich tapestry spread throughout the equatorial regions, with each thread signifying a distinct flavor profile shaped by the local climate, geography, and agricultural techniques. These areas are more than isolated bits of land; they are the cradles of some of the most cherished and unique coffee beans, all adding to the world's harmonious blend of tastes that fans adore.

The Arabica coffee plant grows well in Ethiopia's high-altitude regions, frequently recognized as the country where coffee originated. Ethiopian coffee is consumed ceremonially and is more than just a beverage; it's a trip through old traditions. Ethiopian coffee is well known for its wide variety of flavors, ranging from Sidamo's robust and earthy undertones to the wine-like acidity of Yirgacheffe. Coffee from Ethiopia has a unique wildness to it that adventure-seeking consumers love. This is a result of the country's unique terroir.

When one travels to South America, the coffee landscapes of Costa Rica, Brazil, and Colombia present a distinct, yet no less alluring, image. Colombia produces coffee renowned for its moderate sweetness and well-balanced acidity due to its diversified topography and excellent climate. With coffee estates dotted around the verdant slopes, Colombian coffee culture is intrinsic to the nation's identity. Conversely, Brazil is the world's largest producer of coffee, with its expansive plantations producing beans with a rich, nutty flavor. On the other hand, higher altitude-grown Costa Rican coffee is praised for its vibrant acidity and zesty undertones, which attest to the nation's dedication to excellence.

As one ventures into the volcanic soils of Central America, Guatemala's Antigua area shines out, yielding coffees with a noticeable chocolate undertone and smokiness. Guatemalan coffee is favored by taste enthusiasts who want a symphony of flavor in each cup because of the microclimates the surrounding volcanoes create. Neighboring Honduras and Nicaragua add to the area's diversity by producing coffees with distinct flavors ranging from deep and chocolaty to fruity and sparkling.

After crossing the ocean to Asia, one might find a coffee experience unlike any other in the Indonesian highlands of Sumatra. The Indonesian archipelago offers the perfect growing conditions for Arabica and Robusta beans. Wet-hulled processed Sumatran coffees have a rich body, slight acidity, and a unique earthiness.

The end product is a cup that captures the wild spirit of the verdant surroundings.

Beyond Ethiopia, nations such as Kenya and Tanzania carve out distinct places for themselves on the global coffee map. Because of the country's high altitudes and rich volcanic soils, Kenyan coffee is distinguished by its brilliant acidity, robust body, and vibrant fruity aromas. Tanzania's commitment to quality and sustainability is evident in its variety of coffees, which spans from bright and floral to deep and winey due to its different microclimates.

A trip through coffee-growing regions would only be complete with stopping to explore the beautiful highlands of Mexico's Chiapas region or the high plateaus of Colombia's Sierra Nevada. These areas provide layers of richness to the global coffee landscape by contributing to the rich mosaic of flavors. For example, the Chiapas region is well-known for its Arabica beans cultivated in shadow, which get complex aromas from various plants surrounding the coffee bushes.

As we go through various coffee-growing regions, it becomes clear that each one has a distinct influence on the beans it produces. The interaction of soil makeup, climate, and altitude creates a particular song that reverberates in every cup. Coffee is more than simply a beverage; it's also a form of expression for culture, a narrative about a place, and a sensory excursion through the environments that produce this beloved bean. The next time you enjoy a cup of coffee, think about the trip it took to go from a far-off coffee-growing region to your mug and enjoy the diverse range of aromas that are captured in every sip.

## Roasting Process

An essential step in transforming raw coffee beans into the fragrant concoction that fills our cups every morning is roasting. This transformation process gives the beans their distinct flavors and fragrances and showcases the skill of coffee makers worldwide.

Roasting green coffee beans with heat triggers a chemical reaction that unleashes various flavors and aromas. When green beans are harvested from tropical coffee bushes worldwide, they don't have the typical flavor profile of the full-bodied coffee we love. Thus, roasting serves as the alchemical furnace in which these beans experience a significant metamorphosis.

A complicated chemical reaction occurs in the green beans as heat is applied. The Maillard reaction, named after the French chemist Louis-Camille Maillard, is one of the most important reactions. The formation of the rich brown color of roasted coffee and the synthesis of several taste components result from this reaction between amino acids and lowering sugars in the beans. Roasting beans involves a delicate dance called the Maillard reaction, which requires talent on the part of the roaster to master to create the ideal balance of tastes, from a slight bitterness that gives the cup depth to a sweetness evocative of caramel.

A crucial element in the roasting process is timing. As the beans move through stages indicated by color, aroma, and auditory clues, roasters closely observe them. The first crack, which sounds like popcorn and is a characteristic sound, shows that water vapor and carbon dioxide are being released from the beans. At this crucial point, the roaster stops for a lighter roast or goes on for a darker, bolder profile. This choice significantly impacts the final coffee's flavor, defining whether it will be a fruity, light-bodied Ethiopian or a robust, dark-roasted Italian espresso.

The equipment used for roasting also influences the result. Conventional drum roasters offer a tried-and-true approach akin to big revolving cylinders. Conversely, hot air roasters use a stream of hot air to roast the beans, giving you greater precise control over the process. Because each method adds subtleties, roasters can customize their approach to bring out the best qualities in particular bean kinds.

Beyond the details, roasters are also motivated by a profound respect for the provenance and unique characteristics of the beans they work with. Through their skill, roasters seek to accentuate the unique flavor qualities of single-origin beans derived from specific geographic regions. A Sumatran Mandheling's earthy undertones or the fruity notes of a Kenyan AA—the roasting process is a vehicle through which the natural qualities of the beans are highlighted.

Specialty and artisanal methods have been increasingly important in the recent rebirth of coffee roasting, both an art and science. Small-batch roasters prioritize quality over quantity, are sometimes independent, and have emerged as brand ambassadors for uncommon and distinctive coffee varietals. These roasters support openness in the coffee supply chain by establishing personal connections with coffee growers and guaranteeing just remuneration for their efforts.

Furthermore, roasting is an ongoing pursuit of excellence rather than a static endeavor. Roasters perform a complex dance of trial and error, varying temperature, time, and even the source of the beans to craft specialty blends that satisfy changing consumer tastes. The result is a vivid coffee landscape where connoisseurs may savor a wide range of flavor profiles and learn about the subtleties that contribute to the unique experience of each cup.

To sum up, the roasting procedure is evidence of the alchemy involved in the production of coffee. It is the furnace in which green beans transform into the flavorful, aromatic concoctions we serve on our tables. Roasting embodies a deep respect for the various origins of coffee beans and a dedication to skill, even beyond the minutiae of temperature and duration. Let's appreciate the tastes in every sip of our morning coffee, but let's also recognize the craftsmanship and passion that go into each roasted bean.

# Chapter II

## Essential Coffee Brewing Equipment

### Coffee Makers

When making the ideal cup of coffee, selecting a coffee maker is crucial. Coffee makers come in various shapes and capabilities, each adding to the magic of turning ground coffee beans into a beautiful beverage. They are generally regarded as the unsung heroes of our morning rituals.

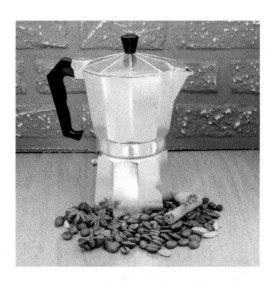

The classic drip coffee machine, a reliable fixture in kitchens everywhere, is the foundation of coffee preparation. These machines are simple to use and always provide a dependable cup of coffee. After heating up, water is poured over a basket containing ground coffee, allowing the scents and flavors to permeate through and be captured. The drip coffee maker is an excellent option for individuals who want a hassle-free, traditional brewing experience because of its simplicity.

The manual pour-over method is considered an artisanal approach to coffee brewing for people who enjoy the sensory experience of creating their coffee. With this technique, hot water is slowly and circularly poured over ground coffee, giving exact control over variables like extraction time and water temperature. The end product is a complex cup that showcases the nuances of the unique coffee beans and the brewer's talent.

The French press, a tool that blends simplicity and potent flavor extraction, has grown in popularity in the wake of specialty coffee culture. After steeping in hot water, coarsely ground coffee is separated using a mesh plunger. The end product is a robust and full-bodied brew that brings out the coffee beans' inherent oils. For those who value a hands-on approach to brewing, the French press allows them to be deeply involved in each process step.

The espresso machine, a marvel for connoisseurs who yearn for the richness and intensity of concentrated coffee, was created with the dawn of contemporary technology. These devices make the famous shot of espresso by applying high pressure and heating water to finely ground coffee. Espresso makers have developed to meet various needs; models range from completely automated ones that simplify the brewing process to manual lever machines that require a deft touch. Beyond the traditional shot, espresso machines can make various popular coffee drinks, such as lattes, cappuccinos, and Americanos.

The single-serve coffee maker is a popular option for those seeking convenience without sacrificing quality. For people with hectic schedules, pod-based systems—like coffee capsules—offer a convenient and mess-free option. These devices, which are frequently fitted with cutting-edge technology, guarantee uniformity in each cup, offering a practical substitute without compromising the flavor of a well-prepared cup of coffee.

The AeroPress, a little, multipurpose gadget that has won over coffee lovers, is a rising star in coffee brewing. This portable device uses air pressure to force hot water through coffee grinds, producing an intense, velvety brew that tastes like espresso. A favorite among travelers and people who value the freedom to try out various brewing methods, the AeroPress is lightweight and straightforward to operate.

Understanding technology's influence on coffee makers' development is crucial as we traverse their varied terrain. With its programmable features and Wi-Fi connectivity, innovative coffee makers have ushered in a new era of unmatched control and personalization. Now, enthusiasts may experiment with pre-infusion settings, schedule brewing periods, and change the temperature of the water—all from the comfort of their smartphones. This technology-coffee craftsmanship marriage allows users to customize their brewing experience to the nth degree.

In summary, a wide range of options are available in the world of coffee makers to suit every taste and inclination. It is a dynamic and expansive terrain. Each method adds to the rich tapestry of coffee culture, be it the simplicity of a drip coffee maker, the tactile artistry of pour-over techniques, the durability of a French press, the intensity of espresso machines, the convenience of single-serve options, or the innovation of gadgets like the AeroPress and innovative coffee makers. Selecting a coffee maker becomes a statement about who we are, how we value and enjoy this age-old beverage, and how we brew it. The variety of choices guarantees that there is a coffee maker that is ideal for every coffee fan, ready to transform every morning routine into an instance of flawless brewing as we set off on our adventure to make coffee.

## Grinders

The primary coffee grinder is a silent hero in coffee crafting, capable of transforming ordinary coffee beans into a flavorful symphony. Grinding coffee is an essential and sometimes overlooked procedure that significantly affects the finished product's flavor, aroma, and overall quality. In this investigation of grinders, we will explore this ostensibly simple device's function and its complexities in the quest for the ideal cup of coffee.

A coffee grinder is a precision tool to grind coffee beans into uniformly sized granules. The power of grinding to enhance flavor extraction in brewing makes it so important. The grinder may be a flexible instrument in the hands of a discriminating coffee connoisseur because different brewing methods call for different grind sizes.

Propeller grinders and burr grinders are the two main categories of grinders. Blade grinders are affordable and generally accessible devices that chop beans with a revolving blade. However, their inconsistent grinding sizes frequently lead to uneven extraction, which changes the flavor profile. Burr grinders, on the other hand, provide a more regulated and personalized grinding experience because of their precisely constructed grinding mechanics. The burrs, which are usually composed of ceramic or metal, grind the beans between them to create uniformly sized particles that enhance the complexity and harmony of a cup of coffee.

Making the primary option to choose a burr grinder or a blade grinder can have a great impact on the quality of your coffee. Coffee experts prefer burr grinders because they can extract the entire range of tastes from the beans, even though they are frequently more expensive. Burr grinders include changeable settings that let users customize the grind size to meet the demands of different brewing techniques. The burr grinder is an adaptable tool for achieving the best possible brewing results, whether you're grinding coarsely for a French press or finely for espresso.

Beyond the finer points of grind size, coffee bean grinders are essential for maintaining freshness. Coffee beans accelerate the oxidation process when ground because they expose a greater surface area to the surrounding air. Because of this, pre-ground coffee frequently lacks the rich characteristics of freshly ground beans. When coffee lovers own a grinder, they can ground their beans right before brewing, guaranteeing that every cup has the maximum flavor and aromatic richness.

It's critical to consider the grinder's speed and uniformity while aiming for the ideal grind. As the oils evaporate during the grinding process, high-speed grinders produce heat that may change the coffee's flavor profile. Slow-speed heroes, on the other hand, especially those that use a burr mechanism, provide a kinder and colder grinding experience, retaining the delicate oils and tastes that characterize each cup of coffee.

As grinders have developed, intelligent technologies have been incorporated, bringing convenience to coffee-making. Users can precisely duplicate their preferred grind size with programmable settings, scheduled grinding, and dosing capabilities, which removes the need for guesswork and improves the brewing experience overall. Grinder technology is at the forefront of innovation, fusing contemporary and tradition as it continues to influence the art of coffee manufacturing.

Grinding is more than just making coffee; it's an art form that lets people customize their coffee experience to suit their tastes. The sensory experience of preparing coffee is enhanced by the physical interaction with the grinder, the aroma generated throughout the grinding process, and the anticipation of tastes just waiting to be revealed. In essence, the grinder is a doorway to the universe inside the coffee bean, where each burr revolution or blade spin brings you one step closer to discovering a symphony of flavors and scents.

To sum up, the grinder represents accuracy, personalization, and freshness and is a doorway to the essence of coffee brewing. Choosing between the accuracy of a burr grinder and the ease of use of a blade grinder shows how dedicated you are to the art and science of coffee production. Allow the grinder to be your ally as you set out to make coffee; it will lead you to the harmonious perfection found in each meticulously ground coffee bean.

## Measuring instruments and scales

When brewing coffee, accuracy is the key to discovering myriad flavors and scents. Unsung heroes, scales, and measurement devices discreetly but considerably improve the quality of the brew. We examine how these tools affect precision, consistency, and, ultimately, the quality of each cup in this examination of their function in the coffee-making process.

Brewing with Precision: A Fine Balance Fundamentally, coffee is a careful balancing act between water and coffee grounds. Scales are helpful in this process of precise measuring needed to reach the ideal equilibrium. The importance of scales is not limited to their measurement capabilities; they guarantee a reliable brew every time. The exact ratio of coffee to water is essential whether making coffee in an espresso machine, French press, or pour-over method. Scales serve as a compass for coffee connoisseurs, helping them navigate the complex world of coffee manufacturing and consistently produce the perfect brew.

Scale Types: From Low-Tech to High-Tech: Coffee lovers have many options when choosing scales. For accurate measurements, essential kitchen scales—which are frequently digital—offer a straightforward yet practical way to measure water and coffee grounds. For many home baristas, these are the workhorses since they are dependable without needless complexity. Conversely, people who want a more participatory and data-driven coffee-making experience are increasingly drawn to high-tech scales with extra features like integrated timers and connectivity to brewing apps. A person's brewing style and desired level of intricacy are often reflected in the scale they choose for their craft.

Regularity in Brewing: The Use of Measuring Instruments A good barista will always be consistent, and measurement equipment is more than just scales—they also include calibrated scoops and measuring spoons. By ensuring that the precise amount of coffee is used for every brew, these gadgets remove the uncertainty that may cause differences in taste and strength. The uniformity attained with these measuring devices is purposefully chosen to respect the integrity of the coffee beans and their distinctive qualities, not only for convenience's sake.

The other component of the equation is water: Although most people use scales to measure coffee grinds, water-measuring equipment is just as necessary. Accurate monitoring of the water's temperature is possible during the heating process thanks to specialized thermometers. Measuring cups guarantee the proper amount of water is added to the coffee maker, preserving the delicate equilibrium necessary for the best extraction. A symphony of flavors is produced by the measured interaction of coffee and water, with each note adding to the overall harmony of the brew.

Beyond Measurable: Harmonizing Art and Science Although exact measures are crucial, the art of brewing coffee cannot be boiled down to a simple scientific formula. Measuring tools are guides that let enthusiasts experiment and get better at what they do- measuring turns into a contemplative practice and a way to connect with the brewing process. Measuring tools enable people to explore while offering a consistent safety net as the coffee world welcomes the union of art and science.

Teaching Resources for Future Baristas: Additionally instructive are scales and measuring devices, particularly for individuals unfamiliar with coffee. Gaining insight into how various ratios affect flavor profiles and extraction times improves one's understanding of the intricate nature of the process. Measuring instruments allow coffee drinkers to experiment with different ratios with precision, which many find enjoyable. With the help of these resources, aspiring baristas can refine their techniques and progressively get an intuitive grasp of the various aspects that affect the finished cup.

The Path to Mastery: Obstacles and Benefits: Although measuring devices are pretty helpful, there are obstacles to perfecting coffee preparation. Novices might need help understanding the subtleties of various beans and the complexities of brewing ratios. But the benefits are well worth the work. The person gets the confidence to brew without the safety net of precise measurements as their expertise increases and the once-measured stages become second nature. An important turning point in becoming an expert coffee maker is moving from a heavy reliance on scales and measuring instruments to a more intuitive approach.

Accuracy as a Route to Excellence: Scales and measuring equipment are the directors in the coffee-making symphony, directing each instrument to play its role precisely. These instruments transform routine tasks into handicraft works, such as measuring coffee grounds precisely and calibrating water temperature. Scales and other measuring devices play an indispensable role in the quest for the ideal cup of coffee, regardless of one's level of precision in measurement or level of intuition in brewing. This equipment stays in style as the coffee community does, guaranteeing that each brew is a tribute to the careful balancing act between art and science in coffee brewing.

## Water Quality

Water quality is a silent but potent orchestrator in coffee perfection, influencing the symphony of flavors that dance in our cups. Although coffee beans justifiably take center stage, water plays an often-underappreciated role in brewing. Water isn't just a way to dissolve coffee grinds; it's the unsung hero that has the power to enhance or detract from the flavor of your beverage.

The capacity of water to function as a solvent and extract the ingredients that give coffee its unique flavor makes it crucial for coffee production. This extraction process is significantly impacted by the chemical makeup of the water, with essential variables being pH level, mineral content, and general purity.

The mineral content of water is one of the main factors to be considered. Although too many minerals can affect the delicate flavor balance in coffee, they contribute to water's overall taste profile. The critical actors are sodium, calcium, and magnesium; their concentrations need to be in the Goldilocks zone, which is between too little and too much. If your coffee has too many minerals, it may taste quite harsh; if it has too few, it may taste bland and lifeless.

The pH of the water is equally crucial since it influences the solubility of coffee components. Coffee water should ideally have a pH of 6.5 to 7.5. Too acidic or alkaline water can cause coffee to be over-extracted or under-extracted, leaving a cup that is overly bitter or lacking depth.

One cannot stress the importance of water cleanliness above and beyond mineral content and pH. Pollutants, smells, or impurities can spoil your coffee's delicate flavors. This is where water filtration plays a crucial but frequently ignored role. Purchasing a premium water filter can significantly improve the water's purity for brewing, guaranteeing that the actual colors of the beans are showcased in your coffee.

Now, let's explore how different brewing techniques are affected by the quality of the water. A typical household appliance, drip coffee makers are sensitive to water hardness. Hard water's mineral buildup can impair the machine's overall function and the heating element. Maintaining the effectiveness of your drip coffee maker and, by extension, the caliber of your brew requires regular descaling.

Conversely, manual brewing techniques, including pour-over and French press, provide greater control but necessitate a deep comprehension of water dynamics. The mineral level can significantly impact the flavor profile of pour-over coffee, as water and coffee grounds interact closely. It's a delicate dance, requiring accuracy in both execution and measurement.

Meanwhile, fans of the French press have to deal with the immersion brewing method. Here, the coffee and water are in contact for an extended period, producing a rich and full-bodied taste. The trick is to locate that sweet spot where the water quality enhances the coffee flavor without being overwhelming.

Espresso is a robust and powerful brew significantly affected by water quality. It is essential to utilize water as pure as possible because the high pressure used in espresso machines amplifies the effects of water contaminants. A slight variation in the water quality can result in an espresso shot that isn't as rich and fragrant as it should be.

It is insufficient to concentrate only on the caliber of your beans or the accuracy of your brewing technique if you want to achieve coffee perfection. The water you use with each sip shapes the aroma and taste that will welcome your senses like an invisible architect. The alchemical medium turns ordinary coffee grounds into an exquisite sensory experience.

The complexity of water quality in coffee production makes it clear that a comprehensive strategy is needed to achieve brewing perfection. It is about realizing how the water and the beans work together harmoniously and recognizing each component's individual roles in the finished product. Think of water as more than just an ingredient; instead, see it as a crucial partner in making coffee that merits our respect and consideration.

Finding the ideal cup of coffee ultimately comes down to striking a balance between the water, the brewing process, and the coffee beans. It's a path that encourages investigation, testing, and a growing sense of gratitude for the alchemy in our kitchens each morning. Thus, remember this as you set out on your coffee-making journey: your water's quality is the silent conductor arranging the harmonious blend of flavors in your cup.

# Chapter III

## The Art of Grinding

### Importance of Grinding

Many consider coffee the drink that awakens people and facilitates intimate encounters, so coffee is a complex concoction that requires accuracy throughout production. The underappreciated hero among the many variables affecting the flavor profile of your brew is the standard coffee grinder. Grinding coffee beans is crucial in creating the ideal cup by allowing the scent and taste to come together.

The primary function of grinding is to turn all the coffee beans into granules that can be extracted. This seemingly insignificant operation is essential because it is based on the fundamental idea that the extraction process is directly impacted by the surface area exposed during grinding. How well water interacts with coffee grinds to extract tastes, aromas, and essential oils depends on the grind's fine or coarse.

The first step in the process is realizing how the brewing method and grind size work in harmony. Various techniques, such as the traditional drip brewer, the complex pour-over, or the sturdy espresso machine, require a particular grind size to maximize extraction. For example, a coarse grind works well for the slow immersion of a French press, resulting in a more robust cup, but a fine grind is essential for the quick extraction needed to make espresso.

Grinding with precision is essential since the incorrect grind size might cause excessive or under-extraction, limiting the cup's potential. A lack of depth and sourness are signs of under-extraction, which happens when the water hasn't had enough time to interact with the coffee grounds. On the other hand, over-extraction, characterized by bitterness and astringency, indicates that the water was left in on unwanted chemicals for an extended period.

Grinding has an impact that goes beyond size; it also affects uniformity. Because smaller particles extract more quickly than larger ones, variations in particle size might result in uneven extraction. The discord in extraction times undermines the harmony desired in a well-balanced cup by producing a brew with a potpourri of flavors. An excellent grinder that can grind coffee beans into uniform particles acts as the conductor of the tastes found in the coffee beans.

In addition, experts place a great value on the freshness of the grind. After being ground, coffee beans quickly lose their volatile components. The aromatic oils that give freshly ground coffee its alluring aroma are susceptible to oxidation. Grinding should preferably occur with brewing to retain the subtle aromas that set apart a genuinely great cup.

Grinding is an art that allows for experimentation and personalization beyond its technical complexities. Coffee lovers frequently take great satisfaction in adjusting the grind size to suit their tastes. The grinder becomes a self-expression tool that lets people customize their brews to perfection, whether the goal is a robust, intense espresso shot or a softer, more subtle pour-over.

Specialty coffee is the domain where varietals and terroir are paramount, and the grinder assumes the role of keeper of each bean's distinct qualities. Only when ground precisely can the complex flavor profile of a single-origin coffee, which is impacted by altitude, soil composition, and climate, be fully expressed. In this instance, the grinder serves as a conduit between the bean's unique characteristics and the drinker's sensory experience.

To sum up, the significance of grinding in preparing coffee goes beyond its technical appearance. Beans change from raw materials to a canvas of flavors ready to be retrieved through this magical gateway. Achieving a superb cup of coffee requires careful consideration of every aspect of grinding, including consistency, freshness, and grind size, to orchestrate a harmonious sensory experience. As you begin your coffee-making adventure, remember that the grinder is more than just a tool—it is the mastermind behind the flavor of your coffee and the silent curator of your daily pleasure in the excellence of brewing.

## Types of Grinders

Grinding is a crucial step in the coffee-making process that creates the delightful transition from whole coffee beans to a cup of coffee. Coffee grinding is an artistic process, and the type of grinder used dramatically influences the final brew's quality and flavor profile. When it comes to choosing a grinder, coffee lovers have a plethora of alternatives, each accommodating a variety of tastes and brewing techniques.

Coffee grinders can be branched into two main categories: burrs and blades. Each has pros and cons of its own. For many coffee lovers, blade grinders—a straightforward design with a rotating edge—are an economical and convenient choice. The ease of use of blade grinders is accompanied by difficulties, though, as it can be challenging to get a constant grind size. Blade grinding's irregular surface frequently produces a mixture of fine and coarse particles, affecting how well flavors are extracted during brewing.

Burr grinders, on the other hand, are the pinnacle of grinding performance because of their exceptional consistency and precision. These coffee grinders consist of two rotating burrs, one fixed and the other adjustable, which grind coffee beans evenly between them. This precise procedure yields a more uniform grind size, essential for bringing out the complex flavors concealed in the beans. Burr grinders are flexible enough to precisely modify the grind size, making them suitable for a variety of brewing techniques, such as French press and espresso.

Two varieties of burr grinders—flat burr grinders and conical burr grinders—further enhance the grinding experience. Burrs on flat burr grinders are oriented horizontally, and they work well to produce a uniform-size grind. Because of this characteristic, they work exceptionally well for espresso brewing, where consistency is crucial. On the other hand, conical burr grinders are known for their capacity to retain less heat during grinding and for operating quietly, thanks to their vertically aligned burrs. This quality helps keep the coffee beans' subtle flavors and scents intact.

When coffee fans explore the world of grinders further, they will likely come across both manual and electric models. Hand grinders are popular among people who enjoy the physical and sentimental aspects of preparing coffee since they are evocative of the old-fashioned hand-cranked mills. Manual grinders, which provide some control over the grinding process, are frequently chosen by individuals who prefer a more hands-on and contemplative approach to brewing coffee. Conversely, electric grinders are the pinnacle of effectiveness and ease. These coffee grinders meet the needs of many busy people by quickly grinding entire beans into a uniform grind at the touch of a button.

There is more to choose from between various kinds of grinders than just blades and burrs, electric and manual. Grind settings, a sometimes disregarded but essential function, allow the coffee fan to customize the grind size to meet the demands of their preferred brewing technique. Espresso requires an excellent grind, so a grinder with exact adjustments is needed for the proper extraction. On the other hand, a coarse grind is essential for techniques like the

French press, where a more porous coffee bed is preferred. Variability in brewing methods and coffee profiles can be explored using a grinder offering various grind settings.

The material makeup of the burrs in the grinder is something to take into account when trying to achieve the ideal cup. The two most common materials are steel and ceramic, each having unique qualities. Steel burrs are solid and practical, and they work well at providing a steady grind over time. They are the go-to option for large-scale coffee grinding because of their robustness. Contrarily, ceramic burrs are well known for their ability to withstand heat, which guarantees that the subtle nuances of the coffee beans are preserved throughout the grinding process. Ceramic burrs appeal to people who value the preservation of subtle flavor notes, even if they could be more brittle.

To sum up, the variety of coffee grinders is equal to the range of tastes they enable. Selecting a coffee grinder is a personal experience, ranging from the tactile engagement of manual alternatives to the efficiency of electric counterparts and from the simplicity of blade grinders to the precision of burr grinders. Knowing the subtle differences between each kind of grinder and factors like burr type and grind settings allows the coffee lover to go on a tasty adventure. The aroma of freshly ground coffee fills the air, a tribute to the importance of selecting the correct grinder—a crucial component in the harmonious combination of ingredients that results in the ideal cup of coffee.

## Grind Size for Different Brewing Methods

The grind size is crucial in creating the ideal cup of coffee, as it can affect flavor, fragrance, and overall brewing success. The proportion of the coffee particles affects the pace of extraction and, in turn, the final brew's flavor profile. The relationship between grind size and brewing method is a complex one.

Let's start with the fundamentals. A crucial component in the brewing equation, the grind size describes how coarse or fine the coffee grounds are. Gaining the ability to modify the grind size by your preferred brewing technique is like having a taste wand; it lets you customize your coffee experience to the fullest.

A coarse grind is essential to bring out the full-bodied richness of cold brew and French press processes. A robust and full cup is produced by the slow extraction method, made possible by the coarseness of the coffee grounds in a French press, which allows the water to mix with the settings without over-extracting. Likewise, a coarse grind for cold brew contributes to a smooth, mellow flavor profile without the bitterness that comes with finer grinds because of the longer steeping time.

Espresso, on the other hand, needs to be ground very finely, almost like powdered sugar. Because espresso machines extract coffee quickly, a finer grind is required to expose the coffee particles' greater surface area more immediately. The strong smells and tastes that are necessary for a balanced and potent shot of espresso are extracted by this fine grind. A coarse grind would cause under-extraction when brewing espresso, providing a weak and dull cup of coffee.

A medium grind is ideal for many homes' drip coffee machines because it provides the perfect balance. This grind size ensures the flavors are extracted consistently by promoting an even extraction over a moderate brewing duration. Going too far in either direction from the medium grind could upset the balance of flavors and cause either an over- or under-extraction.

The pour-over technique requires a medium to medium-fine grind and is praised for its accuracy and capacity to highlight the subtle flavors of specialty beans. The precise amount of water poured over the coffee grinds necessitates a grind size that makes extraction uniform and brings out the unique qualities of the beans. An overly fine grind could produce bitterness, while an excessively coarse ground could produce a sour taste.

Depending on the brewing duration you desire, the Aeropress is a flexible brewing instrument that can hold a variety of grind sizes. When the extraction time is reduced due to a finer grind, the resulting coffee exhibits a more pronounced acidity and brightness in its flavor profile. On the other hand, a smoother, less acidic cup is produced when a coarser grind is combined with a more extended extraction period. Coffee lovers can customize their brew to suit their tastes by experimenting with the grind size thanks to the Aeropress's versatility.

Remember that these are only recommendations; finding the ideal grind is a matter of personal preference. Adjusting the grind size allows you to personalize your brewing experience and make each cup just how you like it. The ideal grind size can be affected by variables including humidity, roast degree, and the provenance of the coffee beans, making coffee-making an art that is both a science and a personal exploration of flavor.

In conclusion, the key to exploring the wide range of flavors coffee offers is comprehending the connection between grind size and brewing techniques. To uncover the subtleties concealed within each coffee bean, you must traverse the landscape between coarseness and fineness, which makes experimentation a crucial ally. The grind size acts as your compass, pointing you toward a perfect cup of coffee, whether you're enjoying a rich French press brew, the intensity of espresso, or the subtle nuances of pour-over.

# Chapter IV

## Mastering Water and Ratios

### Water Temperature

Coffee brewing is a simple process that requires a complex dance of variables, each contributing to your cup's harmonious blend of tastes. Of all these variables, water temperature is a quiet maestro that significantly impacts the finished product. Since water temperature affects the extraction of components that give coffee its flavor, fragrance, and body, mastering the subtleties of water temperature in coffee preparation is like discovering the secrets of flavor alchemy.

When preparing coffee informally, water temperature is a crucial factor that needs to be considered. Coffee can be brewed at a precise temperature, usually between 195°F and 205°F (90°C and 96°C). The magic happens in this temperature range when the solubility of coffee components is maximized and an extraction that is nuanced and well-balanced results.

Those passionate about making the best cup of coffee often need help with whether to use hotter or colder water. It's a complex choice that depends on the preferred flavor profile and the brewing technique. Warmer water, on the more seductive side of the range, tends to remove the chemicals faster, making the cup bolder and possibly stronger. Conversely, colder water—about 195°F—extracts flavors more gradually, resulting in a more delicate and lighter brew.

The effect of water temperature is especially noticeable when comparing various brewing techniques. A higher temperature is typically preferred in drip brewing, where water runs through a bed of coffee grinds. The water captures the flavors contained in the coffee grounds as it filters through, thanks to the higher temperature that guarantees effective extraction. On the other hand, a slightly lower temperature may be used in manual processes such as pour-over or French press, where water interacts with the grounds for a longer duration to provide a gentler extraction and preserve the coffee's characteristics.

The intense and concentrated beverage known as espresso has specific temperature requirements. Espresso extraction is a fast-paced, high-pressure process that requires accuracy. If the temperature is too high, it could force the extraction of unwanted bitter components; if the temperature is too low, the flavors might not have enough depth and richness. To achieve a subtle and well-balanced shot that encapsulates the coffee beans' flavor, espresso connoisseurs frequently strive for water temperatures at the lower end of the ideal range.

In addition to its direct effect on flavor, water temperature is a significant factor in determining how aromatic your coffee will smell. Temperature fluctuations affect the volatile chemicals that give freshly brewed coffee a pleasant smell. The ideal temperature of the water guarantees that these compounds are released into the atmosphere, producing an aroma that enhances the overall pleasure of the drink.

It's important to remember that there is no one-size-fits-all method for getting the ideal water temperature. Altitude, humidity, and the kind of coffee beans used can all affect the perfect temperature for brewing. The boiling point of water is mainly affected by size, necessitating adjustments to account for changes in air pressure. Coffee preparation is an art form that goes beyond science. Therefore, experimentation and a sharp palate are valuable tools in pursuing the ideal brew.

Understanding the interdependence of all brewing variables is essential as we traverse the nuances of water temperature in coffee production. A precise dance between temperature, coffee-to-water ratio, and grind size determines the final composition of your cup. The secret to understanding the alchemy of flavor is consistency in these components, enabling you to duplicate and improve your favorite brew precisely.

To sum up, water temperature plays a masterful role in the coffee-making symphony, guiding the extraction process that turns ordinary beans into a drink with extraordinary intricacy. Coffee lovers may take their brewing game to the next level and produce cups that genuinely capture the artistry of the brewer by learning to embrace the subtleties of temperature and how it interacts with other elements. When you set out on your next journey to make coffee, remember that temperature is more than simply a measurement in the world of coffee; it's the key to unlocking the entire range of flavors each expertly produced cup offers.

## Coffee-to-Water Ratios

The delicate dance between coffee and water—a symphony of flavors and scents that culminate in a sensory delight—is the secret to making the ideal cup of coffee. To unlock the full power of your coffee beans, you must grasp the seemingly straightforward concept of the coffee-to-water ratio to achieve this harmonious equilibrium.

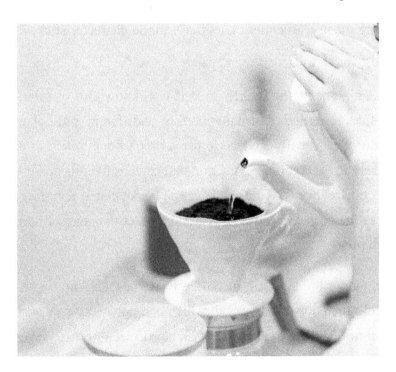

Fundamentally, the ratio of coffee grounds to water used during brewing is what is meant to be understood by the term "coffee-to-water." Even though this seems like a simple calculation, it significantly affects the finished cup. A brew that deviates even little from the ideal ratio risks being unsatisfactorily weak and bland or excessively bitter and spicy.

To properly traverse this terrain, one must first understand how closely the brewing method affects the ratio selection. Each technique—drip coffee, French press, pour-over, or espresso—needs a different balance to extract the desired tastes. For example, the widely used drip coffee method usually requires a ratio of one to two: one part water to one part coffee. When this ratio is used regularly, the result is a cup that balances strength and subtlety, enabling the user to enjoy the coffee's subtle characteristics without bitterness.

On the other hand, the French press is well-known for its robust and flavorful brew, and it usually prefers a different ratio. For this procedure, it's usually advised to use a ratio of one to fifteen or one to sixteen to get a robust extraction that catches the oils and essence of the coffee beans. The coarse grind necessitates a higher ratio because the coffee grounds have a more extensive surface area in a French press.

The equation for the ratio of coffee to water takes on a new level thanks to the pour-over method, which is renowned for its accuracy and control. Here, a percentage of one to fifteen or one to seventeen works best because it strikes a compromise between the necessity for a well-rounded flavor profile and the gradual, regulated extraction process. Pour-over connoisseurs frequently play around with little ratio tweaks, tailoring it to their tastes and the unique qualities of the coffee beans.

Because of its potent and concentrated flavor profile, the world of espresso requires a unique method when it comes to ratios. Espresso is typically made using a ratio of one part coffee to two parts water. But to get the perfect espresso shot, you have to be precise about everything, from the amount of the grind to the pressure at which you tamp it. The slightest variation in the ratio of coffee to water can determine the difference between a great shot and a mediocre one.

Knowing the factors affecting the ratio is just as important as knowing the precise proportions of each brewing technique. Various factors, including the freshness of the coffee beans, the water temperature, and the size of the grind, influence the delicate equilibrium. Specifically, the grind size plays a co-conductor role in this symphony, affecting the pace of extraction and, in turn, the optimal ratio of coffee to water.

Experimentation becomes a valuable ally in the quest for brewing perfection. Since everyone has different tastes, one person may find the perfect ratio different from another's. Discovering the ideal ratio of coffee to water is an adventure you should embark on with an open mind, your taste buds, and a willingness to adjust the parameters to your preference.

Consistency and precision are the keys to mastering the coffee-to-water ratio, just like in any other culinary technique. Purchasing a trustworthy scale to weigh the water and coffee grinds will guarantee that every cup accurately reflects your selected ratio. This dedication to accuracy helps you become a better brewer and makes it possible to make the ideal cup consistently.

To sum up, the key to creating fantastic coffee is the coffee-to-water ratio. The compass leads the coffee brewer through the vast and fragrant world of coffee, providing the chance to customize each cup to personal tastes. Elevate your coffee-making skills by accepting the subtleties of this ratio, comprehending its significance in various brewing techniques, and trying to discover the ideal balance. As you embark on this adventure, remember that finding the perfect cup is as much about the journey as the final product—a journey driven by the desire to take that elusive, transcendent sip.

## Importance of Consistency

A genuinely excellent coffee experience is built on consistency, an art that goes beyond the limits of brewing. The importance of consistency in a world where coffee culture has developed into a dynamic tapestry of flavors and brewing methods cannot be emphasized. Every sip reflects a dedication to perfection rather than just a technicality.

Fundamentally, consistency ensures that each cup of coffee accurately reflects the chosen blend, brewing technique, and individual preferences. When all the components of producing coffee come together in perfect harmony, a sensory experience that is dependable and satisfying is paid for. This consistency is essential for individuals with refined palates who want a known and reliable flavor profile with each brew.

A commitment to quality and consistency begins with the choice of coffee beans. The beans are the starting point for the whole coffee-making process, whether from the lush plantations of Colombia or the high-altitude terrains of Ethiopia. Maintaining consistency necessitates a steadfast dedication to choosing the best beans possible, considering variables like origin, variety, and roast level. The coffee maker creates a steady foundation for the tastes that will eventually dance on the taste buds of the coffee enthusiast by upholding a consistent standard in bean selection.

Achieving consistency also requires careful consideration of the grinding process. The rate at which tastes are released during brewing largely depends on the size of the coffee grinds. For a homogeneous extraction and, thus, a consistent flavor profile, consistency in grind size is crucial. To fully extract the flavor and potential of the selected coffee beans, grinding to a precise consistency is essential, whether you choose a chunky grind for a French press or a drip grind for espresso.

The ratio of water to coffee is a crucial factor that emphasizes maintaining uniformity when brewing. A cup that does not successfully capture the required tastes can occur from even a tiny deviation from the suggested ratio, which can cause either over- or under-extraction. Meticulous measurement practices guarantee that the brewing process continues to be a dependable means of imparting the complex flavors of the coffee beans. Thus, maintaining ratio consistency becomes essential to achieving a consistently enjoyable cup.

Its impact also extends to the brewing technique used. Whatever one's preference—the pour-over method's accuracy or a French press's immersion method—mastering the selected process demonstrates a commitment to a reliable brewing experience. Every technique has its subtleties, and the skilled coffee maker knows how important it is to follow these details. Maintaining consistency in the brewing process turns it into a ritual: a series of intentional steps that provide an excellent and dependable cup of coffee when followed to the letter.

The area where consistency has the most significant impact is temperature management. Every degree of water temperature affects the final flavor profile and substantially impacts the extraction process. Ensuring preserving the delicate balance of acidity, sweetness, and bitterness requires consistency in maintaining the proper temperature. Temperature constancy is crucial in either brewing a robust dark roast or a delicate light roast; it protects the intended range of flavors.

For the seasoned coffee connoisseur, the quest for consistency is broader than the technical aspects of brewing. It includes the process's ceremonial components. The whole experience is enhanced by maintaining consistency in the morning routine, selecting the ideal brewing hour, and even the setting where coffee is consumed. The everyday routine becomes a ritual, a sequence of actions that pays off with a reliably delicious cup of coffee at the end.

Experimentation is another area where consistency is crucial. Variety may be the flavor of life, but consistency acts as the coffee maker's compass as it navigates the wide world of options. The coffee lover can adjust factors while preserving a baseline of dependability thanks to the anchor, which permits controlled exploration. Consequently, consistency becomes the blank canvas that allows for the expression of creativity without sacrificing the quality of a well-brewed cup.

Beyond the sphere of personal fulfillment, sharing the skill of coffee manufacturing with others is profoundly affected by consistency. Building a loyal customer base is a commitment for coffee shops and other enterprises. Replicating the same outstanding cup every day encourages customer loyalty and trust. A cup of coffee can be transformed from an occasional treat to a dependable friend via consistency, forging a connection between the coffee maker and the coffee lover.

In conclusion, it is impossible to exaggerate the value of uniformity when brewing coffee. The thread creates a tapestry of flavor and satisfaction by interlacing the complex components of bean selection, grinding, brewing, and personal ritual. Maintaining consistency is a means to maximizing each coffee bean's potential rather than a hindrance. It's a pledge made to the drinker and oneself that every cup will be a harmonious fusion of tastes that consistently captures the essence of the selected blend. In the ever-changing world of coffee culture, consistency is the age-old secret to flawless brewing.

# *Chapter V*

## Classic Brewing Methods

### Drip Coffee

Drip coffee, celebrated as the ideal morning drink, embodies simplicity in a world of intricate brewing techniques. Its widespread use in homes and coffee shops attests to its enduring appeal and reassuring routine. Making drip coffee is as simple as it is satisfying: water and ground coffee combine in a slow, rhythmic descent to release the flavors and fragrances that characterize a daily awakening.

The combination of premium coffee beans and exact brewing makes drip coffee unique. The amount of water in coffee, the size of the grind, and the type of beans used significantly impact the final result. Coffee lovers can experiment with various settings on drip coffee makers, ranging from manual pour-over devices to electric machines, to create a personalized brew that suits their tastes.

Drip coffee's appeal is due to its simplicity as well as its versatility in a range of environments. The classic drip coffee maker, frequently a kitchen fixture, easily accommodates the morning rush and provides a consistent cup with little effort. When used by a knowledgeable barista, manual pour-over techniques turn brewing into a sensory experience, with each pour and bloom adding to the evolving symphony of flavors.

Investigating coffee beans is the first step towards comprehending the subtleties of drip coffee. The final brew is influenced by the roast character, freshness, and selection of single-origin and blend beans. With every cup, single-origin beans, prized for capturing the distinct terroir of a particular area, take drinkers on a voyage throughout the coffee globe. Conversely, blends—created with great care to harmonize the flavors—offer a smooth, steady flavor that appeals to individuals who want to taste the same every time they sip.

The grind size is another crucial aspect in the drip coffee equation that determines how quickly the coffee is extracted during brewing. While a finer grind speeds up the extraction process and produces a more robust, powerful cup, a coarser grind allows for a slower extraction, giving the coffee a subtle, mild flavor. Coffee lovers can customize their drinks to suit their tastes by navigating the range of grind sizes, which turns a morning routine into a ritual.

While the coffee beans and grind size lays the groundwork, the water-to-coffee ratio acts as the conductor, arranging the tastes into a harmonious whole. Reaching the optimal ratio guarantees a harmony between intensity and complexity, keeping the beer from going too thin or harsh. This is where accuracy is crucial. Whether measured methodically or intuitively, the secret to perfect drip coffee is identifying the sweet spot that appeals to each person's taste buds.

The ease of use and uniformity that characterize a drip coffee maker are enhanced by its mechanics, ranging from a complex automatic machine to a traditional pour-over cone. A more hands-on and reflective approach to brewing is made possible in a pour-over situation, where the slow, deliberate pouring of hot water over the coffee grinds permits a regulated extraction. Instead, because they automate the process, drip coffee makers are vital in hectic homes and busy coffee businesses where productivity is paramount.

The process investigates sensual delight from bean to cup rather than technical details. The intangible aspects that transform drip coffee from a simple beverage to a treasured experience include:

- The aroma that permeates the air when hot water meets coffee grinds.

- The anticipation that grows with every drip.

- The rich hue gradually fills the carafe.

The versatility of drip coffee goes beyond how it is prepared; it also works well with different coffee cultures. It represents the morning routine, a calm moment before the day begins, or a companion to the newspaper in Western societies. In the East, especially in areas such as Japan, the painstaking pour-over method is considered an artistic endeavor, with a ritual that celebrates the process of brewing as much as the final product.

Drip Coffee's continued success in the ever-changing coffee landscape is a testament to its egalitarian nature. It appeals to both the novice coffee user looking for a comforting cup and the expert wanting to explore the subtleties of flavor. Its adaptability makes it a staple of coffee culture that endures the test of shifting tastes and fads. Its versatility surpasses the limits of time and trends.

Drip coffee's understated yet profound essence is like an empty canvas, ready to be adorned with flavor. It invites coffee lovers to explore the comforts of their homes or the atmosphere of a nearby coffee shop, whether served with the elegance of a dash of milk or enjoyed unadulterated. The soothing trickle contains not just a morning ritual but also a timeless reminder that perfection in brewing is rooted in simplicity.

## French Press

The French Press, often known as the press pot, is still a well-known and classic way to brew coffee. People adore it for how easy it is to use and how much taste each cup has. The design dates back to the late 19th century and originated in France. It has stood the test of time and is now a standard in homes and coffee shops worldwide. The capacity of the French Press to extract strong tastes and fragrant oils makes it stand out and appeals to those who want a more involved approach to their brew.

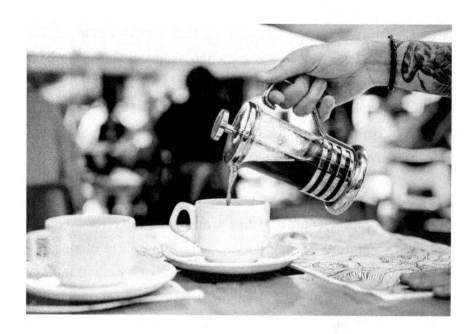

The French Press's basic design consists of a cylindrical glass or stainless steel container, a mesh-filtered plunger, and a lid. But this ease of use conceals the complexity of learning the skill of French Press brewing. Hot water is introduced to the press after coarsely ground coffee beans have been inserted. The magic happens when the coffee and water combine to create a rich, robust brew during the steeping time.

Immersion brewing is emphasized in the French Press, one of its distinguishing features. In contrast to drip systems, which depend on water trickling through the grounds, the French Press promotes prolonged contact between the coffee and water. The long steeping time, usually four minutes or more, permits flavors that could be lost in faster brewing techniques to be extracted. Consequently, you get a cup of coffee that perfectly captures the flavor profile of each bean.

When making French press coffee, the grind's coarseness is crucial. A finer grind could result in a murky and bitter cup. Therefore, a coarse grind is necessary to avoid over-extraction. The balanced extraction produced by the coarse grind and long steeping period highlights the coffee's inherent sweetness and complexity. Because of this harmony, the French Press is an excellent option for highlighting the subtleties of single-origin coffee, allowing the unique scents and flavors to come through without being overpowering.

A metal mesh filter is another essential component of the French Press that adds to the coffee's robust texture. Unlike paper filters that absorb oils, the mesh in drip systems lets oils pass through, giving the coffee a smooth and sumptuous mouthfeel. Those who enjoy the strength and richness of a genuinely great cup will value this distinctive feature.

The French Press provides a medium for delving into the complexities of coffee, but it also necessitates close attention to detail. One crucial factor is the temperature of the water. The optimal temperature range is 195°F to 205°F because hotter water might burn the coffee beans and make them bitter. Reaching the ideal water-to-coffee ratio is equally important; too little coffee might make a weak and dull cup, while too much coffee can make an overpowering brew.

Beyond the details, there is a ritualistic element to brewing coffee that the French Press epitomizes. Pushing down the plunger and watching as water and coffee are transformed into a liquid artwork is a physical and visceral sensation. This manual approach makes an intimate involvement in every step of the brewing process possible, which welcomes engagement with the process from grind size to pour.

The French Press's usefulness goes beyond making black coffee the traditional way. It provides a framework for artistic investigation, allowing for different augmentations and modifications. Experimenting with the brew time can deepen flavors for those who prefer a more robust cup, while others can add spices or flavored syrups. The French press is also a gateway to cold brew since its design allows for the prolonged steeping necessary for smooth and concentrated cold coffee extraction.

Regarding coffee preparation, the French Press is a monument to the union of elegance and simplicity. Its capacity to encapsulate coffee in its most basic form accounts for its ongoing appeal. The French Press offers a trip beyond the simple act of brewing, from the aromatic bloom that occurs when hot water meets freshly ground beans to the satisfying press that creates a liquid symphony in the cup. It's a declaration that sometimes the deepest joys come from the most straightforward approaches and a celebration of artistry and the bean.

## Pour-Over

In coffee connoisseurship, the pour-over method is a highly regarded blend of flavor and accuracy, and achieving the ideal cup is considered an artistic endeavor. The simplicity and mastery of this manual brewing method have made it popular among coffee lovers worldwide. Pour-over started as a Japanese technique called "manual drip." Still, it has developed into a ritual that goes beyond simple brewing. It is a contemplative procedure that extracts subtle flavors and provides a sensory experience that no other way can match.

The basic idea behind the pour-over method is to pour hot water over coffee grounds, usually contained in a cone-shaped filter, in a constant and regulated stream. What appears to be a simple procedure is a careful balancing act involving time, coffee, and water. The elegance of pour-over coffee is in its capacity to highlight the distinctive qualities of the coffee beans, giving the consumer a chance to fully appreciate the range of tastes found in the selected mix.

The degree of control pour-over offers the brewer is one of the main characteristics that distinguishes it. You can fine-tune every aspect, such as water temperature and the way you pour, to achieve the specific results you're aiming for. With this much control, a coffee lover may become a real alchemist, adjusting factors to bring out the ideal body, acidity, and sweetness in the coffee grinds.

Freshly ground coffee is usually used to start the pour-over procedure, which preserves the volatile components in the beans for a more colorful and fragrant cup. An important consideration that affects the extraction rate and, in the end, determines the flavor character is the grind size. The bloom, which is the captivating release of carbon dioxide as the coffee grounds mix with the water and mark the beginning of flavor extraction, happens when the hot water is poured over the grounds in a circular motion.

The key to successful pour-over brewing is timing. The slow pour, frequently made possible by a kettle with a narrow nozzle, enables the water to react with the coffee grounds at a rate the coffee maker sets. This timing creates a sensory experience akin to a dance between coffee and water that turns an ordinary chore into a healing ritual.

The equipment selection further defines the pour-over experience. Different pour-over equipment, such as the Hario V60, Kalita Wave, and Chemex, each contribute a distinct flavor to the brew. The filters are also critical since they affect the body and clarity of the coffee. For example, metal filters let more oils pass through, adding to a fuller-bodied brew, while paper filters absorb oils, leaving behind a clean and bright cup.

The soluble components that are extracted by the water as it passes through the coffee grinds add to the finished flavor. The extraction process is affected by the water's temperature, which should ideally be between 195 and 205 degrees Fahrenheit. If the coffee is too hot, it could taste harsh; if it's too cold, it might taste flat. It takes accuracy and knowledge of the distinct qualities of the coffee beans to achieve the ideal balance.

Patience is necessary when brewing a pour-over, and it's frequently rewarded with a cup of exceptional quality. A delicate extraction that highlights the subtleties of single-origin beans or the harmonic blending of a well-chosen blend is made possible by the slow, meticulous procedure. This leisurely technique emphasizes the journey as much as the destination, in contrast to the quick pleasure of modern coffee machines.

Beyond its technical aspects, the pour-over method is charming because it reflects a thoughtful connection to the brewing process. The rise and fall of the coffee bed, the perfume filling the room, and the visual poetry of water meeting coffee grounds all become subtle shifts that the brewer becomes aware of. The pour-over process elevates brewing to an art form in this small-scale endeavor, demanding skill and a sincere love for the trade.

A well-done pour-over yields a cup of coffee that showcases the flavor of the beans and the brewer's artistic ability. Now freed from the restrictions of mechanized machinery, the tastes dance over the palate, varying in intensity based on the brewer's skill and the chosen beans: bright and acidic, rich and full-bodied, or subtly subtle. Every drink becomes an adventure, investigating the subtleties that make coffee a fascinating beverage.

Beyond its deliciousness, pour-over brewing has come to represent a return to handcrafted quality in the coffee industry. Coffee enthusiasts are encouraged to slow down and enjoy the process using the pour-over method, even when convenience frequently wins out. It creates a community of enthusiasts who value the creative process as much as the final product.

To summarize, pour-over coffee production celebrates skill and an endeavor to create the ideal cup rather than just a brewing technique. Every stage of the pour-over process, from the deliberate bean selection to the captivating pour and the patient wait for the brew to finish, adds to a ritual that turns brewing coffee into an artistic endeavor. When you set out on your pour-over adventure, remember that the secret is not only in the ingredients but also in the careful symphony of flavor and accuracy that can be created in the comforts of your home through the cautious dance of water and coffee.

# Chapter VI

## Advanced Brewing Techniques

### Aero Press

The AeroPress has become a revolutionary icon in the ever-evolving world of coffee brewing, completely changing how aficionados approach their daily routine. Designed by Alan Adler in 2005, this simple plastic gadget has a devoted fan base because of its capacity to brew a cup of coffee that perfectly balances simplicity and precision. In contrast to conventional brewing methods, the AeroPress method offers a unique blend of immersion and pressure, resulting in a cup that captures the entire range of flavors contained in the coffee grinds.

The AeroPress is a cylindrical apparatus comprising a chamber and a plunger. Its clever mechanics and straightforward design let the magic happen. When making coffee with the AeroPress, the grounds are added to a paper or metal filter at the bottom of the brewing chamber. Hot water is poured over the grounds, and the coffee is extracted using the plunger's air pressure. Travelers, coffee lovers, and even professional baristas love AeroPress because of its ability to remove rich tastes from seemingly simple ingredients.

The adaptability of the AeroPress is one of its essential characteristics. In contrast to conventional brewing techniques, which frequently call for precise measurements and specific grind sizes, the AeroPress is flexible and forgiving. Because it can handle different grind sizes, it's a flexible option for people needing access to a high-precision grinder. Users can explore and customize the procedure to suit their tastes, thanks to the freedom offered by adjusting the brewing time and water temperature. The AeroPress may provide a longer, gentler cup or a short, powerful espresso-style shot, depending on your preferences.

The AeroPress brewing method's immersion feature facilitates a complete flavor extraction by allowing the coffee grinds to steep in hot water. The rich and complex flavor is produced in the cup due to immersion and air pressure during extraction. The coffee grounds and water are evenly contacted by the plunger's mild stress, which reduces the possibility of over-extraction—a typical mistake with several other brewing techniques—and encourages an even extraction.

Users of AeroPress frequently talk about how special it is to produce a concentration of coffee that can be used as the base for a wide range of drinks. This concentrate can be used as the foundation for lattes, cappuccinos, and even iced coffee, or it can be diluted with hot water for a regular cup of coffee. With just one small gadget, the AeroPress can satisfy a wide range of tastes and preferences, making it a coffee lover's equivalent of a Swiss Army knife.

The AeroPress is unique in the fast-paced world of contemporary coffee consumption because of its quickness. Because the brewing process can be completed in minutes, it's an excellent option for people who value quality over efficiency. The AeroPress makes dependable coffee in a quarter of the time it takes to make traditional techniques, whether you're a morning commuter looking for a quick yet delicious cup or a traveler missing home.

The quality of the coffee beans is crucial for any brewing method, and the AeroPress is no different. Because the tool brings out the flavors of the beans, it is essential, to begin with premium, freshly ground coffee. The size of the grind still matters; for best extraction, a medium to fine grind is frequently advised. This focus on high-quality, freshly sourced ingredients highlights AeroPress's dedication to providing an exceptional coffee experience.

Beyond its helpful features, AeroPress has fostered an enthusiastic user base that shares skills and recipes and competes internationally. Every year, fans worldwide get together for the World AeroPress Championship, highlighting the inventiveness and commitment of individuals who have adopted this brewing technique. The AeroPress community provides evidence of the device's ability to innovate within a simple procedure, as seen by their creative approaches and the variety of water-to-coffee ratios they have tried.

The AeroPress has been increasingly popular among professional settings, home brewers, and coffee enthusiasts. Baristas have started using AeroPress to highlight the subtle nuances of particular coffee beans in specialty coffee shops and competitions. Because of its mobility, affordability, and ease of use, coffee professionals who want to showcase their selected brews' distinctive qualities will find it a compelling option.

Beyond only its physical appearance, the AeroPress has changed how coffee is made, which has a significant impact on the coffee business. Its emphasis on speed, adaptability, and simplicity casts doubt on the idea that excellent coffee demands sophisticated equipment or labor-intensive procedures. When coffee is brewed with an AeroPress, it becomes a simple and pleasurable experience that encourages experimentation and strengthens the bond between the maker and their cup.

AeroPress has proven to be a revolutionary tool in the coffee industry. Due to its versatile coffee-making capabilities and straightforward yet clever design, this machine has won over the hearts of coffee lovers worldwide. The AeroPress proves that coffee can be made to perfection using a simple yet revolutionary gadget, as seen by its modest origins in 2005 and the widespread praise it continues to receive today. Thus, the AeroPress allows you to discover the art and science of brewing—a trip that starts with a straightforward plunge and finishes with a rich, flavorful cup of coffee- regardless of your experience as a barista or interest in coffee consumption.

## Siphon Brewing

In the world of coffee brewing, siphon brewing is an intriguing demonstration of science and artistry, with techniques ranging from the conventional to the cutting edge. This 19th-century technique, often called vacuum or siphon brewing, is still used today because it makes a perfect cup of coffee. Its popularity in the coffee world is evidence of this. Siphon brewing is a complex process combining aesthetics and physics elements to provide a visually stunning and palate-pleasing theatrical experience.

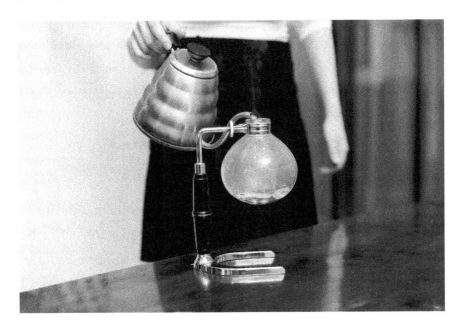

The core of siphon brewing is a gadget with two chambers connected by a tube and looks like a lab experiment. Coffee grinds are in the upper chamber, and water is kept in the lower chamber. Vapor pressure causes the heated water in the bottom chamber to ascend into the upper chamber, where it combines with the coffee grounds. The brewed coffee is returned to the bottom chamber, filtered, and served when the heat is turned off. More than just a brewing technique, this intricate dance of water and coffee turns the process of brewing coffee into a captivating show.

The choice of coffee beans is the first step in the siphon brewing process. The process brings out the subtleties of flavor; thus, selecting the right beans becomes essential. In the siphon, single-origin beans or expertly blended blends take center stage. Each variety promises a unique profile that the process is ready to extract and highlight.

The grind size used for siphon brewing is different; it is finer than what is suggested for a French press but coarser than that used for espresso. This medium grind makes proper extraction possible During the brewing process. The careful grinding prepares the ground for the delicate choreography that occurs when coffee grounds and water come together.

The siphon brewing apparatus is a complex combination of metal, glass, and occasionally fabric filters. Unquestionably visually appealing, the device is a glass globe held over an open flame or halogen heater, giving it the appearance of a tiny chemical experiment. Beyond appearance, the design has a practical use. A cleaner cup is produced when the brewed coffee is drawn back through the filter by the vacuum effect produced by the cooling vapor in the upper chamber.

The key to successful siphon brewing is temperature control. To guarantee the best extraction possible without scorching the coffee, the water must be heated to a particular temperature, usually between 195 and 205 degrees Fahrenheit. By controlling the temperature and utilizing a distinct extraction procedure, siphon brewing brings out flavors frequently missed by other techniques. Depending on the beans and the brewer's skill, the end product is a cup of coffee that embodies a spectrum of tastes, from light and floral to deep and nuanced.

Brewing is a sensory process in and of itself. The lower chamber's water boils up to produce an enthralling visual spectacle. The upper chamber's coffee grinds get saturated with vapor as it rises through the tube. The coffee grounds' interaction with the hot water during this flowering phase releases aromatic molecules that create a fragrant prelude to the main act. The entire blending of the coffee and water during the immersion phase facilitates a complete extraction of flavors. Observing the coffee dance in the upper chamber is a celebration of the skill of brewing coffee as much as an anticipation of the outcome.

The ability of the siphon brewing process to yield a complex and full-bodied cup of coffee is frequently lauded. The vacuum effect separates the coffee grounds from the finished cup, which draws the brewed coffee back through the filter, producing a clear, sediment-free beverage. Instead of paper filters, use a cloth or metal filter to enhance the entire sensory experience and add to the rich mouthfeel of the coffee by letting oils pass through.

Siphon brewing has an unquestionable theatricality that transcends its technical aspects. Viewers may see how water and coffee are transformed into superior beverages because of the clarity of the glass chambers. Siphon brewing is elevated from a simple technique to a performance by the sight of vapor rising, the gentle bubbling, and the rich color of the brewed coffee. An immersive experience is created.

Siphon brewing is not for the faint of heart; it takes patience and a certain amount of talent. The method requires meticulous attention to detail, from the size of the grind to the rate at which it is poured, and individuals who are not used to more complex brewing methods may find the learning curve daunting. But the benefits are unmatched for those who are prepared to put in the time and work: a cup of coffee that goes beyond the typical and invites the user to savor a symphony of flavors with each sip.

The return of siphon brewing in modern coffee culture demonstrates the human interest in fusing science and beauty. Siphon Brewing encourages coffee lovers to take their time, interact with the process, and enjoy the finished product at a time when convenience frequently wins out. With this technique, preparing coffee becomes more than just a daily chore; it becomes an artistic endeavor.

To sum up, siphon brewing offers an enthralling exploration of the core of coffee alchemy. Every component of a brewing method—from the carefully selected beans to the complex apparatus and the captivating brewing process—contributes to a technique that is equally about the journey and the destination. A visual spectacle, a symphony of tastes, and a celebration of accuracy, siphon brewing elevates the simple act of producing coffee to the status of an art form. Remember that every cup you brew with a siphon is a work of art simply waiting to be brewed and enjoyed. This will help you on your siphon brewing journey.

## Cold Brew

An excellent and refreshing contender in the ever-changing world of coffee culture, Cold Brew has captured the palates of coffee lovers all over the world. Cold Brew has cemented its position as a differentiated method, providing a distinct and velvety coffee experience that sets it apart from its heated competitors. It is no longer a fad. This elegant, chilled symphony of coffee is more than a passing craze; it's a revolutionary method of brewing that has completely changed how we think about enjoying coffee.

Cold Brew is a way to extract coffee that takes a long time—12 to 24 hours—to soak coarsely ground coffee beans in cold or room temperature water. Cold Brew is a slower brewing method that allows the coffee grounds to release their aromas gradually into the water. It produces a more potent brew than standard hot brewing methods, which use heat to speed up the extraction process.

The secret to Cold Brew's charm is its capacity to yield coffee, a marked contrast to its hot equivalents. For many who find standard iced coffee too strong, Cold Brew is an enticing option because of its smoother, less acidic taste, resulting from the more extended steeping period. The drink gains richness and depth from the lengthy extraction and a canvas of flavors that may be paired with a wide range of inventive additions or savored on their own.

The adaptability of Cold Brew is one of its distinguishing qualities. It tastes excellent simply over ice, but its intense flavor offers up a world of alternatives. Tailoring Cold Brew to personal tastes in terms of flavor and strength is possible by diluting it with water, milk, or a dairy substitute. Furthermore, Cold Brew is a fantastic foundation for creating specialized coffee drinks. It may be painted with flavors, syrups, and unusual garnishes by a creative barista or home brewer.

Although the process of producing Cold Brew is surprisingly easy, it does require careful attention to detail. It's crucial to start with premium, coarsely ground coffee beans. The coarse grind guarantees a slow and even extraction by preventing the over-extraction that might result in bitterness. The coffee bean type is also essential; single-origin beans with distinctive flavor profiles work best in Cold Brew, bringing out the best in each final cup.

Another essential component of the Cold Brew method is the steeping vessel. Although you can use any container, Mason jars, French presses, and specialty Cold Brew coffee makers are the most common options. For optimal saturation and extraction, it is essential to have a vessel large enough to hold the water and coffee grinds. When it comes to Cold Brew brewing, patience is vital. The longer steeping time turns a water and coffee grind mixture into a concentrated potion.

The coffee grinds are usually removed from the Cold Brew concentrate by filtering it once the steeping procedure is finished. The resultant liquid is a potent elixir ready to drink whenever you want and keeps well in the refrigerator. One of the benefits of Cold Brew is its ease; it offers a rich coffee concentration that can be customized and diluted to the drinker's liking.

The popularity of Cold Brew led to a boom in the availability of Cold Brew products that are ready to drink. The same intense and smooth Cold Brew experience may be had with these canned or bottled beverages without requiring any at-home preparation. This change in customer behavior is a reflection of the need for a quick, refreshing coffee choice that fits in with today's busy schedules.

In addition to its sensory appeal, Cold Brew has come to represent innovation in the coffee business. Its popularity is consistent with a significant movement to investigate non-traditional drip or espresso brewing techniques. Various cold coffee options, such as flash-chilled coffee and nitro cold Brew, have been made possible by the growing popularity of cold Brew. Each offers a unique take on the chilled coffee experience.

The benefits of Cold Brew go beyond just flavor; it also has health benefits. Cold Brew is a milder choice for people with sensitive stomachs or acid reflux problems due to its lower acidity. Because of this, Cold Brew is now a well-liked option for anyone looking for a luxurious yet health-conscious cup of coffee.

The culture of specialty cafés and coffee shops has influenced the development of Cold Brew. After being a specialty item, Cold Brew taps have become a mainstay on coffee shop menus, joining drip brewers and espresso equipment. Cold Brew's presentation and serving techniques are as creative as the beverage itself. The visual appeal of Cold Brew elevates the overall experience with sophisticated ice cubes and fashionable glassware.

Even though Cold Brew has made a name for itself as a significant force in the coffee industry, it is still developing. The Cold Brew sector is lively and dynamic due to the research of flavor infusions, utilization of specialty coffee beans, and unusual brewing processes. The appeal of Cold Brew is not limited to its present level of popularity; it also extends to its capacity for ongoing invention and adjustment to suit the ever-evolving tastes of coffee connoisseurs.

To sum up, Cold Brew reflects the changing face of coffee culture rather than just a cold cup of coffee. A break from tradition and embracing a fresh approach to enjoying coffee, Cold Brew is distinguished by its careful brewing method and the whole, velvety aromas it produces. As we raise our glasses to this elegantly cooled symphony, we celebrate not just a cool drink but also a movement in culture that encourages us to discover, try, and enjoy the countless benefits that coffee, in all its forms, has to offer.

# Chapter VII

## Flavored Coffee Creations

### Infusions and Flavored Syrups

In the dynamic world of coffee culture, where creativity and heritage collide, flavored syrups and infusions have become sophisticated accompaniments to the traditional cup of joe. Coffee purists may contend that the purity of the bean contains the genuine essence of coffee. Still, adding complimentary flavors opens new options and elevates the commonplace to the remarkable. This book explores the world of flavored syrups and infusions, showing how these additives enhance coffee preparation's flavor, aroma, and creative possibilities.

The knowledge that coffee, like any culinary art, can be a canvas for various complex flavors lies at the core of our investigation. The method of infusions, steeping coffee with extra ingredients, has gained popularity as a fascinating way to enhance the drink's flavor profile. Inputs give a spectrum of options to play with and reinvent the coffee experience, whether it's the warmth of spices, the sweetness of fruits, or the depth of herbs.

The choice of complementary ingredients is the first step in the infusion process. Cloves, cardamom, and cinnamon can give the coffee a deep, aromatic flavor. Herbs like lavender or mint provide a herbaceous and refreshing complexity, while fruits like berries or citrus peels add a vivid sweetness. Combining these ingredients with coffee results in a fusion that enhances the sensory experience.

Spiced coffee mixes represent one of the most well-known infusion methods. Combining spices like cloves, nutmeg, and cinnamon with coffee is a long-standing custom in many cultures. When these spices are brewed with coffee grounds, the result is a fragrant drink infused with the spices' comforting, warming qualities. As a result, the cup invites the user into a realm of sensual delight and goes beyond the typical.

Conversely, flavored syrups provide a more straightforward and adaptable method of adding flavors to coffee. These syrups act as vehicles for various tastes and are usually created from a foundation of sugar and water. Flavored syrups provide an easy method to customize coffee to suit individual preferences, ranging from traditional flavors like vanilla and caramel to more unusual options like hazelnut or coconut. The coffee world has embraced this personalization, as adjusting each component to one's tastes is often part of pursuing the ideal cup.

Flavored syrups are versatile since they may be easily included in various coffee preparations and offer multiple flavors. Whether it's a simple drip coffee, a luxurious latte, or a refreshing iced tea, flavored syrups play the role of alchemists, transforming the mundane into something delightfully novel. In addition, the practice of making flavored syrups at home has grown in acceptance, giving connoisseurs the freedom to try different combinations and find a harmony that suits their palates.

Supporters contend that adding flavored components is a development that broadens the coffee's flavor profile to accommodate a broader range of tastes, even though some may see it as a departure from the purity of coffee. This progression aims to offer a diverse experience that attracts a broader audience rather than simply masking the inherent flavor of coffee.

The growth of specialty coffee shops and artisanal roasters has greatly aided the popularity of flavored syrups and infusions. Baristas, frequently considered contemporary coffee artisans, play around with unusual pairings, transforming the coffee counter into a flavor-exploring playground. In addition to increasing consumer demand for premium, exotic beans, this trend has also given rise to a culture in which a cup of coffee is a carefully chosen experience.

In the realm of coffee, infusions, and flavored syrups have evolved into storytelling tools in addition to sensory delight. Once a modest drink, coffee now tells stories of faraway places with its infusion of spices from far-off marketplaces or the delicate flavor of fruits from sun-drenched orchards. With each sip, this narrative element invites the coffee drinker to go on a trip, enriching the ritual of consuming coffee.

The addition of tastes to coffee is also in line with the changing culinary scene, which embraces fusion and experimentation. Coffee is now used as a versatile component in cooking, moving beyond its original use as a morning pick-me-up. The possibilities with coffee are endless, ranging from savory dishes with coffee as a secret ingredient to desserts with coffee infusions.

Like other culinary techniques, balance is essential for infusions and flavored syrups. The idea is to enhance and complement the coffee's inherent qualities rather than overpower it. The skill is striking the right balance so that the extra flavors improve the coffee without destroying its natural flavor. Carefully examining the coffee beans utilized, the tastes selected, and the brewing technique is necessary to achieve this delicate balance.

In conclusion, using flavored syrups and infusions in coffee preparation represents a vibrant nexus of innovation and tradition. While the infusion method dates back to antiquated customs surrounding spiced coffees, flavored syrups provide the coffee experience with a modern, adaptable twist. Together, they invite those who enjoy coffee to delve deeper, try new things, and customize their experience. In the constantly changing realm of coffee culture, introducing various flavors broadens the possibilities of what coffee maybe and encourages creativity, storytelling, and a sense of community. We honor the richness and diversity that infusions and flavored syrups provide to the craft of coffee manufacturing as we lift our cups to this union of flavors.

## Spice Blends

Adding spices to coffee is like practicing creative alchemy in coffee's vast and fragrant world, where every cup is a canvas ready to be painted with taste. The custom of incorporating spice blends into coffee transcends national boundaries and transforms the mundane process of brewing into a sensual encounter.

This infusion enhances the coffee's flavor profile and adds depth, warmth, and complexity, enticing coffee enthusiasts to try flavors different than their favorite beans. The history of spiced coffee dates back hundreds of years, and other cultural influences have produced a wide range of recipes that reflect the unique flavors and spices of different regions.

Middle Eastern societies have been producing cardamom-infused coffee for generations. It gives the beverage an intense floral and citrus flavor, making it a daily luxury and a sign of welcome.

Meanwhile, one of the best examples of combining coffee with spices is the well-known "Masala Chai" in India. At the same time, traditional South Indian filter coffee also benefits from a fragrant spice combination.

Making coffee requires careful consideration of the spices you use. The natural richness of some coffee beans is complemented by the popular addition of cinnamon, which has warm, sweet undertones. The earthy, somewhat sweet flavor of nutmeg adds another layer of complexity, and the hint of spice and depth from cloves completes the picture. Because of its fragrant and lemony properties, cardamom is a versatile spice that can counteract coffee's acidity. Ginger, frequently used in chai mixes, adds a spicy and energizing component.

The union of spices and coffee is more than taste; it's a subtle ballet of fragrances that starts when coffee beans touch the grinder. A symphony of aromas is released while grinding coffee with whole spices, setting the stage for the subsequent sensory experience. The heat generated during the brewing process releases volatile oils from the herbs, which combine with the coffee to create a smooth and flavorful combination that entices the senses before the first sip.

Regarding coffee laced with spices, brewing techniques become a creative blank. The pour-over method subtly extracts coffee and spice aromas because of its exact control over water temperature and pouring procedure. Fans of the French press can enjoy the full-bodied flavor of the spices because the immersion method produces a deeper infusion. Because of the pressure-driven extraction process used by espresso machines, robust spice flavors can blend in with the strong coffee flavor.

The process of creating coffee with spices is centered around experimentation. Coffee aficionados become unofficial alchemists, adjusting ratios and combinations of spices until they find the ideal balance that pleases their palates. The secret is to follow a recipe and recognize how coffee beans and herbs work together to create a harmonious flavor profile that lets each component take center stage.

Spiced coffee has global cultural importance that extends beyond the kitchen. In a tradition known as "Bunna," green coffee beans are roasted along with spices like cinnamon and cloves in Ethiopia, the birthplace of coffee. This tradition fosters community and shared experiences while giving the coffee unique scents. The centuries-old Turkish coffee preparation practice of adding cardamom demonstrates a cultural appreciation for Turkey's fusion of innovation and tradition.

The allure of coffee flavored with spices goes beyond following conventional form. Baristas in contemporary coffee shops are experimenting with novel spice blends to push the limits of flavor profiles. These innovations, which range from cayenne-spiced espresso to turmeric lattes, upend preconceived ideas about what coffee maybe and entice a new generation of coffee lovers to experience a world of surprising and daring flavors.

Recognizing the flavors different spices provide to the brew and the potential health advantages of doing so as we traverse the complex world of spice-infused coffee is essential. For example, cinnamon is well known for its antioxidant qualities and possible anti-inflammatory benefits. Cardamom has been associated with better digestive health and breath freshening, while ginger is well known for its digestive advantages.

Still, there's more to the appeal of spiced coffee than just the breakdown of flavors and health advent ages. It appeals to our sentimental and nostalgic parts, bringing back memories of warm winter nights, joyous occasions, or a grandmother's welcoming kitchen. Coffee's fragrant spice blend has a mystical quality that elevates it beyond hydration to a sensory experience that awakens the spirit.

In summary, using spice blends in coffee preparation is an homage to the variety and inventiveness of the coffee industry. Through a sensory journey, fans are invited to discover the diverse sensations offered by various spices, fostering understanding between other nations, customs, and palates. Spice-infused coffee reflects the essence of coffee production as an art. It is ready to be painted with the rich, aromatic hues of spices and coffee beans, whether traditional recipes or cutting-edge inventions inspire it. Thus, enjoy not just the flavors but also the histories and customs that have woven this vicious tapestry of flavor as you set out on your spice-infused coffee journey.

## Creative Additions

In the coffee culture's dynamic field, connoisseurs will come to a new phase of exploration and creativity. A new generation of coffee enthusiasts is pushing the limits of flavor, texture, and presentation beyond the classic black cup of joe. This essay delves into "Creative Additions in Coffee Making," wherein the mundane process of making coffee is transformed into an artistic manifestation, enabling individuals to customize their coffee experience to suit their specific preferences and interests.

There is much room for creativity when preparing coffee; one of the most fascinating areas is experimenting with different flavors. Coffee cups are starting to contain various cutting-edge additives in addition to the traditional sugar and cream. Nutmeg, cinnamon, and cardamom may add depth and warmth, turning a mundane coffee break into a sensory experience. For those who prefer their coffee sweet, adding vanilla extract, caramel, or even a tiny amount of maple syrup brings a welcome sweetness that balances the coffee's natural bitterness.

Coffee lovers now have an arsenal of infusions at their disposal. Adding citrus peels or experimenting with herbs like thyme or rosemary opens up a world of flavor options. These understated touches add layers of depth, transforming a plain cup of coffee into a fragrant experience that appeals to the sense of smell and taste.

The world of spirits and liqueurs has become a playground for coffee exploration for those looking for a riskier enterprise. A lively dimension can be added to the brew by adding a measure of flavored vodka, a splash of whiskey, or even a hint of liqueur. In addition to celebrating the long history of coffee in cocktails— classics like the Espresso Martini having paved the way for more inventive creations—the pairing of coffee and alcohol is a monument to artistic flair.

The inclusion of other milk options expands the canvas even more. The selection of non-dairy milks has increased dramatically, ranging from oat and almond to coconut and macadamia, offering a blank canvas for creating customized coffee concoctions. These substitutes can satisfy lactose intolerances and offer unique tastes and textures that accentuate or contrast with the coffee foundation.

Butter coffee, called Bulletproof coffee, has become increasingly popular recently. This non-traditional addition promises a creamy, frothy beverage with claimed health advantages by combining coffee with grass-fed butter and medium-chain triglyceride (MCT) oil. Although some traditionalists might object to this inclusion, they will try new things to create a unique and decadent cup of coffee.

Coffee's visual attractiveness has also become a central theme for imaginative modifications. Once the purview of expert baristas only, latte art has made its way into residential kitchens. Coffee aficionados share their artistic skills on social media, turning the delicate dance of pouring frothed milk onto the coffee top to create elaborate patterns into a form of self-expression. Ambitious artists have elevated latte art and the clichés of ferns and hearts, producing intricate designs that rival seasoned painters.

The investigation of inventive additives in coffee preparation goes beyond the cup to include coffee- and sweets. Coffee and the culinary arts have come together to create a variety of mouthwatering treats, like espresso-flavored chocolates, coffee-infused ice creams, and coffee-infused tiramisu. These dishes not only satisfy sweet tooths but also demonstrate how adaptable coffee is as an ingredient in a variety of cooking applications.

The third-wave coffee movement and the emergence of specialty coffee shops have been crucial in popularizing innovative additives. These places, frequently managed by enthusiastic baristas, act as testing grounds for new tastes, exposing customers to inventive blends and encouraging a DIY coffee culture. With rosemary-infused cold brews and lavender lattes, these coffee businesses inspire patrons to venture beyond their comfort zones and relish the unusual.

Recognizing the historical and cultural influences that have led to this creative rebirth is crucial as coffee-making develops into a customized and artistic activity. The variety of coffee traditions worldwide, ranging from the solid cardamom-spiked Turkish coffee to the sweetened condensed milk-heavy Vietnamese iced coffee, accentuates the wide range of tastes that can be incorporated into the coffee-making process. In essence, these additions are a tribute to the global history of coffee, beckoning connoisseurs to set out on a flavor-filled, cross-border adventure.

To sum up, innovative approaches to coffee preparation offer a vibrant and fascinating new frontier in coffee culture. Beyond the confines of traditional brewing, connoisseurs embrace a range of tastes, feels, and visuals that elevate the everyday ritual to an artistic experience. The creative possibilities are as varied as the people who create them, whether it's the infusion of spices, the pairing of coffee with spirits, the investigation of substitute milk, or the beauty of latte designs. The only limit to coffee discovery in this day and age is the imagination, with each cup serving as a blank canvas for creativity, self-expression, and the sheer delight of the masterfully crafted original blend.

# Chapter VIII

## Perfecting the Espresso

### Espresso Basics

Within the coffee industry, every brewing technique reveals a distinct story of taste, scent, and customs; espresso is a solid and focused main character. Espresso is a sophisticated blend of science and creativity that has won the hearts and palates of coffee lovers for years. It's more than just a strong jolt of caffeine.

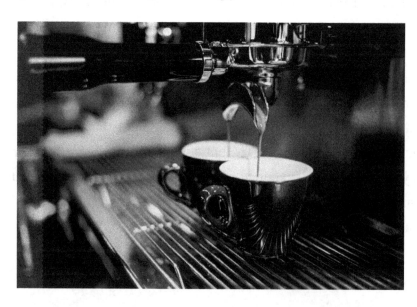

Espresso is a coffee extraction technique that requires applying high pressure and hot water to finely ground coffee. What was the outcome? This potent elixir is characterized by a rich body, velvety crema, and a flavor profile ranging from sharp and bitter to sweet and complex. Although the word "espresso" may conjure up visions of modern machinery and busy Italian cafés, knowing the fundamentals of this brewing process reveals a universe of variables and methods that go into making liquid gold.

The coffee beans themselves are the first step in creating the ideal espresso. Espresso requires very finely ground coffee, similar to powdered sugar, in contrast to other brewing techniques where various grind sizes may be appropriate. Capturing the subtleties of the coffee requires an even extraction of tastes during the short time the coffee is in contact with water, which is made possible by this tiny grind.

The coffee mix is the next crucial component. Arabica and Robusta beans are frequently used in traditional espresso blends, each offering distinct qualities. Robusta provides body and consistency to the crema, while Arabica adds richness and acidity. Several important factors, including the origin, roasting profile, and choice of beans, shape the ultimate flavor profile of espresso.

After laying the groundwork, the actual brewing process takes center stage. The workhorses of this technique, espresso machines, come in various designs, from fully automated marvels that serve the bustling coffee shop to manual lever machines that require a skillful hand. Water, pressure, and time are the three fundamental principles that never change, no matter how complicated the engine gets.

Nine bars of pressure push water boiled to 195 and 205 degrees Fahrenheit through the finely ground coffee. Espresso brewing is known for its high pressure, quickly removing flavors and compounds. Espresso is brewed differently from other coffees due to its short contact time, emphasizing intensity and concentration. This period is usually between 25 and 30 seconds.

A well-brewed espresso is distinguished by its crema, a golden layer of foamy bubbles atop the shot. This crema is a tactile sign of a successful extraction and a visual treat. The crema, made up of oils, proteins, and sugars, captures the coffee's fleeting smells and fragrances and provides a mouthwatering preview of the liquid beneath.

The idea of "tiger striping," a visual indication throughout the extraction process, is introduced by comprehending the role of crema. A balanced extraction is indicated by alternating light and dark bands in the crema as the espresso pours. If you extract too quickly, the bars might be primarily light, suggesting under-extraction; if you pull too slowly, the bands might be too dark, indicating over-extraction. Espresso mastery is found in this delicate tango between grind size, duration, and pressure.

Espresso has a flavor profile, a mosaic of flavors that harmoniously interact, including sweetness, acidity, bitterness, and body. Frequently misinterpreted, bitterness is an essential element that counterbalances the coffee's sweetness. A harmonious blend of tastes is produced by a well-balanced espresso, where the bitterness enhances the entire complexity rather than taking center stage on the palate.

But espresso is more than simply a drink by itself. From the traditional Americano (espresso diluted with hot water) to the smooth and velvety latte (espresso with steamed milk) and the strong cortado (espresso with a tiny amount of warm milk), it forms the basis for a wide variety of popular coffee drinks. Every derivative enhances the espresso foundation, offering a variety of adaptable and customized coffee experiences.

The barista's role becomes paramount in the quest for espresso perfection. A good barista is not just someone who knows how to operate the machine and grind beans; they also have a natural sense of how to steam milk and handle beans. The skill of the craft is in its capacity to change parameters quickly and to discern the nuances of every shot.

Espresso's intense intensity has become a common symbol for a quick pick-me-up, but its cultural significance goes beyond just caffeine. Drinking an espresso at a busy bar is a tradition that breaks up the day in Italy, where the beverage originated. Espresso's cultural significance has spread throughout coffee cultures, elevating the humble brewing technique to a refinement and interpersonal ties symbol.

It's essential to note how the coffee industry is changing as we explore the subtleties of espresso. Espresso is enjoying a revival because of the popularity of specialty coffee, which emphasizes single-origin beans, exact brewing instructions, and a rejection of the one-size-fits-all method. Espresso has evolved from a simple caffeine fix to a sensory experience that highlights the distinctive characteristics of each bean as a result of this change.

In summary, the world of espresso is an intriguing fusion of craftsmanship and science. Every stage of the process, from the careful bean selection to the high-pressure magic of the espresso machine, goes into producing a beverage larger than its tiny size. Espresso is more than just a shot of caffeine; it's an exploration of the flavor profile of coffee, one image at a time, that will reveal, appreciate, and savor a symphony of flavors.

## Espresso Machines

In the world of coffee, the espresso machine is considered an icon—a beloved tool that transforms ordinary coffee beans into a liquid symphony of flavor and perfume. The espresso machine, which has its roots in the busy cafes of Italy, is now an essential part of the coffee culture, providing a doorway to a world where passion, pressure, and accuracy come together. This paper investigates the complex world of espresso makers, going into their background, the technology that fuels them, and the creativity that characterizes the quest for the ideal shot.

The espresso machine originated in the 19th century when engineers and inventors envisioned a device that could extract coffee at a speed and intensity never before seen. However, the early models lacked the finesse found in contemporary espresso makers. The first identifiable espresso machine wasn't patented until 1901, at the very beginning of the 20th century, by Luigi Bezzera. This seminal event set the stage for a gadget that would completely change how we perceive and value coffee.

The alchemical process that transforms coffee grinds into the rich, concentrated beverage known as espresso is at the core of every espresso machine. The underlying idea is simple: a short, powerful shot that perfectly encapsulates the essence of the coffee is produced by forcing hot, pressured water through finely-ground coffee. Nonetheless, the idea's ease of application masks its complex implementation.

The ability of the espresso machine to drive water through coffee grounds at a pressure far higher than that of traditional brewing methods is one of its distinguishing characteristics. Most commercial equipment has a pressure range of 9 to 15 bars, commonly measured in bars. Because of the tremendous pressure, the coffee's aromas and oils are extracted quickly, producing a robust and fragrant brew.

There are many different kinds of espresso machines, each with unique subtleties and qualities. The most common type is the manual machines, in which the barista manages the extraction procedure all the way through. An iconic piece from the past, lever machines represent this group. Sem semi-automatic devices provide a compromise, which automates some steps of the extraction process while retaining some degree of control. Fully automatic devices, which start the whole brewing process with a single button push, are at the other extreme of the range. These varied devices serve a range of coffee lovers, from the hands-on crafter to the convenience-seeking connoisseur.

Modern espresso makers are equipped with technology that is a technical marvel, combining science and art. The boiler is an essential part that heats water to the exact temperature needed for extraction. High-end models are known for having dual-boiler machines, which enable simultaneous brewing and steaming and provide ideal temperature control for both operations. The heat exchanger is another innovation that eliminates the need for two separate boilers to regulate temperature consistently.

When creating espresso, the way the coffee beans are ground is crucial. For the proper extraction to occur, the beans must be coarsely ground to generate resistance. Because of its reliability, burr grinders are favored in the world of espresso. The grind size, expressed in microns, is a crucial factor affecting the espresso's flavor profile and extraction time.

Portafilters, the containers that store the coffee grounds during extraction, are another component of espresso machines. The portafilter's material and design, whether single or double, can affect the flow rate and heat retention, affecting the product in the cup. The coffee bean type determines the complexity of the espresso's flavor, whether they are a single origin or a blend.

The majesty of the espresso machine lies not only in its extraction mechanics but also in its drama of crema, which is the golden layer of emulsified oils that adorns a perfectly drawn shot. Crema is a visual and tactile cue that an espresso was made correctly, so it's more than just a beautiful beverage. The precise amount of pressure during extraction, freshly roasted beans, and the right grind size are all necessary to achieve the ideal crema.

Preparing espresso becomes much more intricate when one learns to tamp or force coffee grinds into the portafilter. A skilled barista applies consistent pressure to guarantee an even extraction. In pursuing the ideal shot, tamping—often compared to an artist's brushstroke on a canvas—is a necessary technical skill and a means of personal expression.

A crucial component of the espresso experience, steaming expands the machine's potential even further. A thin arm that extends from the device is called a steam wand, which froths and warms milk to produce the velvety microfoam necessary for drinks like lattes and cappuccinos. Achieving the perfect texture and temperature involves a careful balance between heat and aeration, so mastering the art of steaming takes skill.

The development of espresso machines has influenced coffee consumption's social and cultural context and technological aspects. Once associated with Italian cafés, espresso has gained worldwide recognition as specialty coffee shops and coffee connoisseurs discover and appreciate this potent beverage's subtleties. The espresso machine's standing as a focal point in the quest for coffee perfection has been further enhanced by the emergence of third-wave coffee culture, which strongly focuses on artisanal techniques and the enjoyment of single-origin beans.

Additionally, espresso machines have come to represent social interaction and community. Cafes are places where people share moments, ideas, and the simple pleasure of a well-crafted espresso. They are adorned with shiny machines and staffed by knowledgeable baristas. Having an espresso, whether by yourself for reflection or in lively conversation with companions, becomes more than just a drink; it's a ritual, a way to break up the day, and a celebration of fine craftsmanship.

To sum up, the espresso maker is a marvel that combines science and art, turning the menial process of making coffee into a flavorful and precise symphony. The espresso machine has evolved from its modest conception in Italy to its current status as a worldwide symbol of coffee culture, more than just a practical tool. The adventure into the world of espresso is a voyage of discovery, an exploration of flavors, and a celebration of the alchemy that takes place within the limits of a well-crafted machine, regardless of your preference for the manual elegance of a lever machine or the ease of a fully automatic model. Within the coffee industry, the espresso maker is a monument to the human desire for the ideal cup.

## Making Espresso-based Drinks

In the coffee industry, where brewing methods abound, producing espresso-based cocktails is the pinnacle of culinary innovation. With its intense flavor and thick crema, espresso is the basis for many drinks that are now commonplace in cafés and homes worldwide. Making espresso-based drinks is a sophisticated process that calls for a combination of accuracy, inventiveness, and a profound understanding of the alchemical potential of coffee. These drinks can range from the bold simplicity of an espresso shot to the delicate layers of a skillfully prepared cappuccino or latte.

The espresso shot, a powerful, concentrated extraction that serves as the foundation for all espresso-based drinks, is what baristas and coffee connoisseurs use to create their masterpieces. The first step is choosing premium coffee beans, ideally a blend designed specifically for espresso with a well-calibrated acidity, sweetness, and bitterness balance. The grind size is essential because the coffee needs to be finely ground to allow for the quick extraction of flavors during the brief brewing period.

A technical marvel, the espresso machine turns finely ground coffee into a liquid essence that embodies the spirit of the beans. In a few seconds, the water pressure to about 9 bars pushes through the coffee grinds, removing soluble chemicals and oils. The end product is a shot of espresso, a flavorful one-ounce liquid that is quite potent. The espresso's golden layer of emulsified oils and gasses, or crema, is a precursor to the richness ahead and a visual and sensory treat in and of itself.

But espresso is an adaptable base for a wide range of drinks, not a goal in and of itself. The Americano is a straightforward but delicious concoction that uses hot water to lessen the strength of espresso, providing a softer taste without sacrificing flavor. With its dollop of foamy milk, on the other hand, the macchiato achieves a delicate balance between the richness of espresso and the smoothness of milk foam.

The cappuccino becomes a work of beauty when we explore the world of milk-based espresso beverages. Made with equal amounts of espresso, steaming, and foamed milk, the cappuccino displays the barista's talent for creating the ideal balance of flavors and textures. The robustness of the espresso blends perfectly with the smooth microfoam, produced by skilled steaming and frothing, to have a decadent and energizing drink.

Another well-liked member of the espresso family, the latte, uses more steamed milk, giving it a creamier, more muted flavor profile. It invites elaborate latte art designs that showcase the barista's artistry and act as a blank canvas for artistic pursuits. Beyond appearance, the latte represents the pleasing interplay of contrasts between espresso's robustness and steaming milk's embracing comfort.

Regarding decadence, the mocha is a rich combination of chocolate, steamed milk, and espresso. This decadent mixture goes beyond the limits of traditional coffee beverages, satiating both the sweet tooth and the urge for caffeine. Rich chocolate and espresso combine to produce a drink that is opulent yet cozy at the same time.

Espresso-based beverages go beyond the traditional menu to satisfy the changing preferences of a multicultural coffee culture. In equal measure, the espresso and warm milk in the cortado help those looking for a well-balanced but intense flavor. Relatively new to coffee, the flat white delivers a robust yet smooth experience by combining velvety microfoam with double espresso shots.

As we delve more into the world of espresso-based drinks, it becomes clear that creating them requires both skill and imagination. The skill of perfectly foaming milk, the deft dance of flavors in the cup, and the accuracy with which espresso shots are poured all combine to create an extraordinary experience. Baristas, often known as coffee artists, become experts at using the espresso machine as their instrument to create taste symphonies that entice the senses.

It is impossible to emphasize the essential quality ingredients while striving for perfection. Beyond the coffee beans, an espresso-based drink's taste is greatly influenced by the type of milk used. From conventional whole milk to substitutes like almond, soy, or oat milk, each adds its distinct flavor and texture, enabling many personalized creations to meet dietary requirements and personal preferences.

Drinks with espresso as the foundation have additional charm from latte art, a visual representation of the barista's expertise. The beautiful rosettes and heart-shaped patterns grown on the drink's surface demonstrate the level of care and attention that goes into each creation. Beyond aesthetics, latte art represents the devotion to skill and the promise to provide an experience rather than merely a drink.

The menu of espresso-based drinks keeps growing in the era of specialty coffee, with creative blends and regional variations contributing to the rich tapestry of coffee culture. Every culture adds its spin to the craft of espresso-based beverages, enhancing the diversity of coffee worldwide, from the Spanish cortado to the Viennese melange.

As we explore the complex realm of creating drinks with espresso as a base, it becomes clear that the procedure is a culinary expression rather than just a ritual. It connects the dots between science and art, requiring technical know-how yet permitting artistic experimentation. From being a simple piece of equipment, the espresso maker transforms ordinary coffee beans into delicious elixirs.

To sum up, creating beverages with espresso is an experience that goes beyond simply preparing coffee. It creatively represents the union of espresso and other ingredients, a symphony of tastes, textures, and scents. Every creation, whether an intricately layered cappuccino or a straightforward espresso shot, results from meticulous attention to detail and passion. Savoring these drinks allows us to celebrate the commitment of people who, one cup at a time, turn a simple coffee bean into a culinary masterpiece and enjoy its rich flavor.

# Chapter IX

## Art of Milk Frothing

### Frothing Techniques

When it comes to the complex art of creating coffee, where every component plays a part in creating a harmonious blend of flavors, the technique of foaming milk is an essential ability. Beyond its practical use in giving lattes and cappuccinos a creamy texture, milk foaming enhances the sensory experience of drinking coffee. This essay delves into the physics, tools, and procedures involved in creating a velvety delight from a plain cup of coffee by exploring the subtleties of milk foaming.

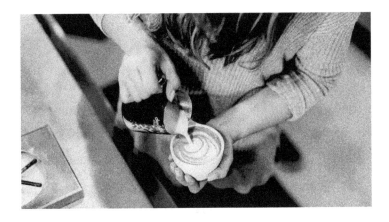

The basic process of milk frothing is adding air to milk to produce microfoam, a soft, velvety foam that rises to the surface of the coffee. The natural proteins in the milk—mostly whey and casein—interact with the air bubbles to create a stable foam, which is when the magic begins. This alteration improves the coffee's texture and adds to its flavor.

The type of milk used is crucial to the foaming process. Because of its high protein content, dairy milk froths up nicely and adds a rich, creamy mouthfeel. But as plant-based milks like almond, soy, and oat milk gain popularity, baristas and home cooks must investigate frothing methods that accommodate these options. Every variety of milk has distinct qualities, so getting the best foam calls for a careful strategy.

The quality and temperature of the milk are critical factors that determine the success of milk foaming. Milk that has been refrigerated is necessary to produce stable microfoam because chilled proteins react with air more efficiently. Nevertheless, the intended outcome determines the optimal temperature for frothing. A warmer milk might work better for lattes, but a colder foam works better for cappuccinos.

While several instruments are available for this task, the most popular ones are handheld frothers and the steam wands found on espresso machines. A standard fixture in coffee establishments, the steam wand is a metal rod that emits pressure steam, giving the frothing process a polished appearance. Using a steam wand to create the ideal microfoam requires expertise and knowledge of the subtleties of the device. However, handheld frothers—which resemble tiny whisks—provide a practical choice for usage at home. Although they lack the steam wand's power, their versatility and ease of use make them a viable option for coffee lovers looking to improve their at-home coffee-making experience.

By placing the steam wand or frother slightly below the surface of the milk, one can introduce air into the milk by the frothing technique. The swirling effect is produced by gradually lowering the frother to submerge the wand as the milk swells. This deliberate movement guarantees that the foam is distributed evenly throughout the milk. Rather than giant, airy foam, the desired texture is a silky microfoam with tiny, velvety bubbles. This difference, which sets a well-frothed latte apart from a mediocre one, calls for a delicate touch on the maker's part.

Beyond selecting equipment, there is an art to achieving the appropriate foam consistency. The amount of air mixed with the milk determines the froth type—dry, medium, or wet. For cappuccinos, dry foam with a higher air content produces a rich, airy feel. While most foam has less air and is better suited for macchiatos, medium foam creates a balance and is perfect for lattes. By being aware of these differences, a barista or do-it-at-home enthusiast can customize the frothing procedure to the exact requirements of the coffee beverage.

A big part of the coffee experience is the texture of the milk foam. Foamed milk should be shiny, silky, and devoid of giant bubbles. The coffee and microfoam should combine to produce a pleasing harmony of tastes and textures. The act of frothing is elevated from an essential technicality to an artistic expression thanks to this attention to detail, where the artistry and expertise of the practitioner influence the final product.

Latte art further elevates the coffee experience by providing a visual representation of the foaming process. Simple hearts, ornate rosettes, and swans are all depicted on the velvety canvas that the microfoam creates. Pouring latte art needs more than just skilled foaming; it also requires a steady hand and an artistic eye. Baristas worldwide have made this a famous and competitive trade component, with tournaments devoted only to the art of lattes.

The foaming process adds to the sensual appeal of coffee and its aesthetic value. The hissing sound of steam produces a multimodal sensation, as do the rhythmic swirling of milk and the olfactory notes generated during foaming. This immersive method gives the ritual of preparing coffee a theatrical touch, whether conducted in the privacy of one's kitchen or witnessed in a busy coffee shop.

Elevated foaming techniques are becoming increasingly in demand as the popularity of specialty coffee rises. Milk frothing is a skill that many who love coffee aspire to learn because they want to replicate café-quality experiences at home. Online guides, courses, and discussion boards have become essential resources, creating a community of enthusiastic people about honing their frothing techniques. The sharing of tricks, troubleshooting assistance, and inventive methods for foaming milk has turned it into a collaborative process of learning and proficiency.

To sum up, milk foaming is a crucial technique that turns a cup of coffee into a sensory marvel. Every aspect of making microfoam, from the type of milk to the equipment, temperature, and frothing technique, adds to the complex process. Beyond its practical use, milk foaming is an artistic medium that lets practitioners customize their coffee drinks' appearance, consistency, and texture. The method of frothing enhances the ritual of preparing coffee, whether in the cozy confines of a home kitchen or a busy coffee shop. It invites connoisseurs to embark on a journey where artistry and accuracy meet, and every sip celebrates skill.

## Creating Latte Art

Latte painting has become a pleasurable and visually beautiful craft in coffee, where presentation is just as important as flavor. Beyond the brewing process, latte art shows off the barista's talent and inventiveness by transforming a plain cup of coffee into a canvas for elaborate patterns and designs. This fascinating custom, which transforms a morning routine into a visual and tactile experience, has come to be associated with the specialty coffee culture.

Latte art is essentially the art of pouring steaming milk into an espresso shot to create visually pleasing patterns on the surface of the coffee. The latte, a coffee beverage with a noteworthy amount of microfoam, serves as the canvas for this artistic expression. Understanding how espresso and milk interact, getting the perfect foam texture, and—above all—learning how to control the milk stream to create elaborate designs are all necessary steps to becoming a latte art expert.

The espresso shot, a concentrated extraction of finely ground coffee beans, is the cornerstone of latte art. The creamy crema of the espresso serves as the canvas's initial layer, and its quality creates the background against which the painting is completed. A photo masterfully composed of smells and scents establishes the mood for the unfolding visual symphony.

The other essential ingredient, steaming milk, provides a canvas for the barista to express their creativity. By adding steam to the milk, the steaming procedure produces microfoam, which gives the coffee a smoother, more velvety mouthfeel. It's an art in and of itself to create the ideal microfoam; it takes careful attention to technique and temperature. If you boil the milk too much, it becomes less sweet; if you heat it too little, the foam won't have the structure needed to create complex patterns.

Learning the fundamental designs of the heart, tulip, and rosette is the first step toward making latte art. The heart is a straightforward yet sophisticated design in which a continuous stream of milk is poured into the middle of the espresso, forming a heart-shaped figure as the milk combines with the crema. The more complex rosette pattern creates a lovely swirling shape that suggests a rose and calls for a gentle side-to-side motion during pouring. The tulip gives the canvas a sophisticated touch with its tiered petals, challenging the barista to control the milk stream's height and flow.

The world of latte art unveils a world of inventiveness and originality beyond these basic motifs. To create one-of-a-kind, customized artwork, baristas experiment with free pour techniques, etching, and even merging different patterns. The canvas turns into an expressive playground, and each cup showcases the artist's talent and creativity.

Latte art is visually appealing, but it does more than look good; it also improves the whole experience of sipping coffee. When the microfoam is expertly blended, it gives the latte a rich, creamy texture that transforms it from a basic drink into a sensory delight. The surface patterns highlight the barista's skill and give the customer a sense of anticipation, enhancing each sip with a hint of surprise and delight.

The third-wave coffee movement, which emphasizes quality, artistry, and the recognition of coffee as an artisanal product, is growing at a rate similar to the advent of latte art. Coffee shops are being transformed into galleries where each cup conveys a different tale by the baristas, who were once marginalized and are now recognized as acclaimed artists. Because of this change in viewpoint, latte art is now more than just a novelty—it represents the coffee industry's dedication to quality.

The making of latte art involves a lot of instruments of the trade. Baristas frequently use narrow-spout stainless steel pitchers to manage the milk flow carefully. The final design is influenced by the tilt of the cup, the angle, height, and speed at which the milk is poured. The plans emerge from the surface tension created by the crema and dairy, and the barista's steady hand acts as a brush to paint the canvas.

Although latte art has come to symbolize specialized coffee culture, its roots are in Italy, where cappuccino art first became well-known. The art form developed and diversified as espresso-based beverages were more widely consumed worldwide, giving rise to distinctive regional styles. For instance, baristas in Japan created cute animals and characters on top of lattes, creating a whimsical and Instagram-worthy scene that quickly gained popularity.

Due to the growing popularity of latte art, baristas can now demonstrate their abilities on a large platform in contests. Artists from all over the world gather for competitions like the World Latte Art Championship, where they compete to be crowned the best latte artist in the world. These contests push the envelope of what is feasible and honor artistic talent, encouraging the next generation of baristas to improve their skills.

Latte art demands patience, practice, and a sincere love for the medium, just like any other art. Baristas set out on a path of constant development, honing their methods and attempting novel designs. The learning process is dynamic, with new opportunities for growth and learning presented by each pour. Latte painting is challenging and exciting because of the unpredictable nature of the canvas, which includes fluctuations in crema, milk temperature, and even air humidity.

To summarize, making latte art combines creativity, talent, and coffee expertise. Coffee becomes a canvas on which baristas may express their love and skill with latte art, ranging from the essential heart and rosette to the intricate tulip. Beyond its aesthetic appeal, latte art elevates the coffee experience, transforming a daily routine into an artistic pleasure. As we enjoy our exquisitely designed lattes, we observe the commitment of the baristas who, one pour at a time, transform a basic brew into a work of art in addition to tasting their skill.

## Milk Alternatives

The milk option for your daily cup of coffee is now wider than whole or skim due to the constantly changing coffee culture. Various milk substitutes have emerged due to changing dietary habits, ethical concerns, and the desire for distinctive flavor characteristics. These dairy-free coffee alternatives—from almond and soy to oat and coconut—have transformed the coffee-drinking experience by providing a diverse range of flavors that suit a variety of palates and lifestyles.

There are several reasons for the rise in popularity of milk substitutes, but the main ones include lactose intolerance, vegetarianism, and environmental concerns. One of the leaders of this revolution, almond milk balances the strength of coffee with a subtle nuttiness and a creamy smoothness. Another early contender is soy milk, which has a neutral flavor profile that lets the natural flavors of the coffee come through while still having a rich, foamy mouthfeel. As these substitutes gained popularity, the industry saw a surge of invention that brought an astounding variety of plant-based milks, each with unique qualities.

The velvety texture and inherent sweetness of oat milk have made it a rising star in the milk substitute arena. Because it froths to perfection, baristas love it, and it improves the presentation of coffee drinks. A wide range of people will like the harmonious combination that the delicate oat flavor creates, which complements the coffee without being overbearing. With its tropical overtones, coconut milk gives coffee a distinctive twist, adding a hint of exotic flair and a creamy richness. For individuals looking to stray from traditional options, coconut milk is popular due to its adaptability, which is evident in hot and cold beverages.

The inclusion of milk substitutes is one of their main benefits. A large percentage of people suffer from lactose intolerance, a common ailment that frequently prevents them from enjoying typical dairy-based coffee beverages. Alternative milk offers a solution, enabling people with dietary constraints to enjoy their morning routines without sacrificing taste or consistency. The need for plant-based solutions has increased due to the growing popularity of veganism; as a result, coffee shops worldwide are now happy to provide a variety of milk replacements to meet the increasing needs of their clientele.

Beyond dietary concerns, a move for sustainable options has been spurred by the environmental impact of dairy production. Customers concerned about the environment have expressed worries about the carbon footprint linked to traditional dairy farming. Milk alternatives made from plants typically have less impact on the environment because they use less water and land. Innovative substitutes offering nutritional advantages and a minor environmental impact, like pea and hemp milk, have been developed in response to the growing demand for environmentally friendly options.

The development of milk substitutes has revolutionized coffee preparation, impacting the final cup's appearance and flavor. Baristas can now experiment with various textures and consistencies instead of being limited to dairy froth. Especially oat milk has proven to be a champion for latte art, creating a velvety microfoam that elevates the aesthetic appeal of coffee concoctions. Professional and home brewers have more options because these substitutes blend well with the specialty coffee industry.

The nutritional quality of milk substitutes offers another level of attraction for the health-conscious consumer. Numerous plant-based alternatives are enhanced with vitamins and minerals, providing an equivalent or even better nutritional value than dairy products. One common technique to address concerns about bone health that may develop with a transition away from dairy is to fortify almond milk with calcium and vitamin D. It's essential to remember that different brands and varieties of milk substitutes have different nutritional values, so consumers are urged to make educated decisions based on their dietary requirements.

Manufacturers are experimenting with a broader range of components and formulas as the market for milk substitutes has experienced a rise in innovation. Various nut milks have emerged, each adding subtleties to the coffee experience: hazelnut milk, cashew milk, and combinations of numerous nut species. These substitutes add to the vast array of options accessible to consumers and provide unique tastes.

There have been difficulties in assimilating milk substitutes into mainstream coffee culture. Some purists contend that traditional dairy products pair best with coffee's distinct flavor and that the abundance of options can compromise the authenticity of the coffee-drinking experience. Concerns over the sustainability of some milk substitutes, especially almond milk, which needs a lot of water to grow, have also spurred discussions about striking a balance between environmental responsibility and customer preferences.

In conclusion, the development of milk substitutes for coffee signifies a fundamental change in how we think about our morning cup of joe. Coffee lovers are no longer limited to the simple decision of cream or milk; instead, they can adapt their experience with a wide range of plant-based choices, each with a unique flavor and texture. Customers can customize their coffee to reflect their views, whether motivated by dietary requirements, moral concerns, or a desire for a more environmentally friendly beverage. The world of coffee is changing, and the dairy-free symphony of flavor reflects that. In the quest for the ideal cup, people around the globe are seeking both innovation and inclusivity.

# Chapter X

## Coffee and Dessert Pairings

### Matching Coffee with Sweet Treats

Few combinations in the complex realm of cuisine can match the classic union of coffee and sweets. For generations, people from many cultures have delighted in the symphony of flavors that arise when the sweetness of cakes, candies, or pastries combines with the bitterness of coffee. This harmonic combination is a delicate balance that requires knowledge of the subtle differences between coffee and sweets; it is not only a question of taste. The skill of pairing coffee with sweets is a quest that enhances the experience, from the bold flavors of dark roast coffee with a chocolate cake to the delicate dance of a fruity Ethiopian coffee with a citrus-infused confection.

The complementing qualities of flavors and textures form the foundation of this delectable combination. Complex components created during the roasting process give coffee its innate bitterness, which balances and intensifies the sweetness of pastries. Each part of the palate symphony that results from this interaction is unique yet harmonious as a whole. To appreciate this culinary skill, one must learn about coffee profiles and investigate how various brewing techniques and bean origins can affect the combination.

A cup of dark roast coffee perfectly matches dark chocolate's rich, complex flavors. The intensity of cocoa and the assertiveness of a Sumatran or Italian roast work together to provide a delightful experience for the senses. A symphony of deliciousness is created when the bittersweet flavors of chocolate blend with the subtle smokiness of the coffee. This traditional combination is a perfect example of the idea that decadent desserts should have equally rich coffee accompaniments.

The subtle nuances of a light roast coffee are highlighted for individuals who prefer fruitier, more delicate desserts. Desserts with berries, citrus, or stone fruits go well with a brightly acidic coffee from Kenya or Ethiopia. The acidity of the fruits and the zesty flavors of the coffee work together to create a palate-pleasing and well-balanced experience. Here, the goal is to highlight and enhance the dessert's sweetness rather than overshadow it.

The brewing process is crucial to nailing the combination, even beyond the broad parameters of roast levels and bean origins. For example, the smooth finish of a well-made espresso pair wonderfully with creamy desserts like cheesecake or tiramisu. With every sip, the concentrated flavors of the espresso cleanse the palette and cut through the dessert's richness. The slow, deliberate pour-over process provides a more nuanced approach, which lets the coffee reveal its layers of taste alongside a skillfully made sweet treat.

Think about the confluence of coffee and pastries, which is cherished in cafés worldwide. A medium roast coffee is the perfect match for a croissant's buttery, flaky layers since the coffee's caramelized sweetness balances the pastry's richness. This combination transcends cultural boundaries and demonstrates the global relationship between coffee and sweet treats.

Examining these combinations must recognize the cultural customs that have influenced how coffee and desserts are consumed. The French art of combining café au lait with a delicate éclair, the Scandinavian tradition of enjoying a cinnamon roll with a cup of coffee, or the Italian routine of sipping espresso alongside a biscotti—all embody the cultural subtleties that have raised these pairings to the status of art.

The coffee and sweet treat combination trip is heavily influenced by personal preferences, much like any other culinary experience. While some people crave the delicate balance of a light roast coffee with a fruit-infused delicacy, others may find happiness in the dramatic contrast of a dark roast coffee with a sweet, caramel-laden dessert. The allure is in the limitless options, which inspire coffee lovers to experiment and create their flavor symphony.

It's important to remember that coffee and sweets complement one other more than taste. The social aspect of appreciating these culinary delights is enhanced by the shared experience of savoring a delightful match. The pairing of coffee and sweet sweets, whether during a festive gathering, a casual talk with friends, or as the focal point of a solitary time, promotes connection and builds enduring memories.

The dynamic and innovative pursuit of pairing coffee with sweet sweets continues in the ever-evolving environment of coffee culture. This culinary heritage fascinates palates and inspires new flavor explorations, from the time-tested classic pairings to the cutting-edge combinations popping up in contemporary eateries. The next time you enjoy anything sweet, think of the symphony of flavors with the ideal cup of coffee. This symphony elevates the commonplace and turns a straightforward action into a moment of culinary genius.

## Coffee in Baking

Beyond the cup, into the fabric of baked goods, coffee appears as a mystical elixir in culinary alchemy, where elements are turned into exquisite creations. Coffee and baking together elevate pastries, cakes, and cookies to new levels of flavor complexity, going beyond the typical morning ritual. The harmonious interplay between the bitter undertones of coffee and the sweet notes of baked goods produces a sensory symphony that appeals to lovers of baked goods and brewed beans.

The adaptability of coffee is the fundamental element of this culinary mix. Its varied taste character, solid and earthy or bright and fruity, gives bakers a wide range of flavors when creating decadent treats. Coffee acts as a silent maestro, arranging flavors to create a symphony that dances on the tongue, whether it's deepening the chocolate flavor of a brownie, giving a hint of bitterness to a sponge cake, or boosting the richness of a creamy tiramisu.

Think about the traditional combination of coffee and chocolate, which goes beyond everyday expectations to produce a marriage of tastes cherished in various baked goods. The sweetness of chocolate and the sharpness of coffee combine to create a pleasing balance that enhances the richness of the chocolate. A chocolate cake with an espresso shot infuses it with a rich flavor that lingers on the palate and creates an unforgettable experience.

Coffee contributes to baked items' texture beyond its flavor improvement role. When coffee is substituted for water or milk in recipes that call for liquids, it adds another level of complexity. Coffee's acidity can react with leavening ingredients like baking soda to give an additional lift that makes the texture lighter and more airy. This transformational effect is most noticeable in baked goods, where coffee is a secret ingredient to achieve the ideal crumb, such as muffins, pancakes, and quick breads.

Coffee enhances flavor in a variety of foods, not only sweets. Coffee gives savory baked items, such as bread and some types of biscuits, a subtle, beneficial depth. Coffee's earthy and mildly bitter flavors can mellow the spicy undertones, providing a well-rounded and captivating flavor profile. This way, coffee crosses the line from sweet to salty, becoming a versatile element in the baker's toolbox.

Additionally, coffee excels as a stand-alone component in various baked goods. Cakes, cupcakes, and cookies with coffee flavors honor the spirit of the beverage, providing coffee enthusiasts with a treat that goes beyond the morning ritual of a cup. The combination of coffee and pastries is most famously displayed in tiramisu, a dessert consisting of layers of creamy mascarpone and ladyfingers soaked in coffee that produce a divine harmony of flavors and textures. Tiramisu is a prime example of how coffee, when thoughtfully included in a dessert, can act as a catalyst, transforming an ordinary confection into a culinary marvel.

Coffee in baking opens up new creative possibilities, especially for frostings and fillings. For example, layer cakes and cupcakes get a refined edge from buttercream flavored with coffee. When the rich, fragrant notes of coffee blend with the velvety smoothness of buttercream, a whole new level of flavor is revealed. This combination results in a frosting that enhances the cake below and serves as a monument to the never-ending research of flavors in the baking industry.

Coffee can be incorporated into less typical recipes in addition to baked foods. Coffee syrups and reductions give typical sweets a gourmet touch. They can be utilized to flavor ice cream or poured over cheesecakes. Desserts with coffee flavorings are becoming more popular, which reflects people's increasing understanding of the complexity of coffee outside of its cup.

Furthermore, "coffee flour" has become popular as a creative method to add coffee to baked goods. This unusual flour, created from ground and dried coffee cherries, gives baked dishes a hint of coffee flavor and an antioxidant boost. Coffee flour's adaptability allows it to play around with recipe ideas and provides a creative approach to adding coffee flavor to a range of baked goods.

Coffee is also used in baking in the artisanal realm of pastries, where talented bakers use its unique flavor to create signature masterpieces. Coffee-infused danishes, tarts, and croissants highlight the careful balancing act between the robust coffee overtones and the buttery layers of pastry. Combining the aromatic essence of coffee with flaky, golden pastry offers a sensory experience beyond the ordinary.

The incorporation of coffee into baking indicates a broader societal shift as the culinary scene develops. It aligns with the trend toward more complex and nuanced palates, moving away from one-dimensional sweetness and toward depth and complexity in flavors. Coffee is the driving force behind this flavor revolution, enabling experienced pastry chefs and inexperienced bakers to push the frontiers of taste with its wide range of scents and tasting notes.

Finally, adding coffee to baking is evidence of the dynamic interaction between two indulgent realms. The sweetness of baked products is complemented by the bitter overtones of coffee, providing a harmonious effect that pleases the senses. The world of baking has embraced coffee as a transforming ingredient, from traditional chocolate pairings to creative experimentation with coffee flour. The combination of coffee and baking is a tribute to the inventiveness and imagination of people who want to take the ordinary and turn it into something spectacular when it comes to food. We can't wait to explore all the unlimited possibilities.

# Chapter XI

## Exploring International Coffee Cultures

### Italian Espresso Culture

A rich and lively espresso culture has taken root in the heart of Italy, where cobblestone alleys reverberate with the footsteps of history and the perfume of freshly ground coffee dances through the air. More than just a drink, Italian espresso is a daily ritual that permeates the ebb and flow of conversation, laughter, and memorable moments in Italian social life. Understanding Italian espresso is like diving into a symphony of custom, ritual, and unrestrained passion that goes beyond the act of brewing.

The espresso, a concentrated coffee extract created by the clever design of the espresso machine, is the fundamental component of Italian espresso culture. The espresso machine, built in Turin in 1884 by Angelo Moriondo, transformed the way coffee was prepared by quickly extracting a tiny, potent shot of coffee. This concentrated elixir served as the cornerstone of Italian espresso, distinguishing it from other brewing techniques and encapsulating the country's philosophy towards coffee.

In Italy, chasing the ideal espresso shot is a kind of art. The first step is choosing premium coffee beans, typically a blend of Robusta and Arabica types. The roasting process is a closely kept secret, as each coffee shop or roastery takes pride in its mix and roast flavor. The end product is finely ground coffee that, when tamped and poured into the espresso maker, produces a velvety crema, or a creamy layer that sits over the espresso and indicates a well-balanced espresso.

Espresso preparation is a sophisticated dance between the barista and the machine rather than just a mechanical procedure. A good barista is aware of the subtleties of grind size, the significance of tamping pressure, and the exact duration of extraction. It's like watching a master conduct a symphony when you watch an experienced Italian barista in action. Every step is calculated to produce the ideal result—a shot of espresso that perfectly captures the flavor of the beans and the barista's skill.

Beyond the coffee, espresso culture is a fundamental part of Italian culture. The Italian "caffe," or espresso bar, is a meeting place for people from many walks of life. It's about community, connection, and enjoying moments together—it's not just about the coffee fix. A place where business deals are closed, friends are made, and the fabric of Italian life is sewn one cup at a time is the espresso bar.

In Italy, placing an espresso order is a craft unto itself. Ordering a "caffè" in Italian espresso culture means getting a shot of espresso according to unwritten standards. Instead of being overly watered down, the coffee's intensity is a concentrated taste explosion that tantalizes the senses. The routine also includes deciding when to have an espresso: as a midmorning snack, after a meal, or as a pick-me-up in the afternoon. Every moment has meaning, and the Italian way of life is reflected in the timing of when to enjoy this little but potent drink.

Espresso consumption is a sensory experience. The rich and nuanced flavor profile, the aroma, and the cup's warmth in your hands all combine to create an indulgent moment. Espresso needs to be taken more seriously in Italy; it is a time to stop, taste, and recognize the skill that goes into each cup. The Italian expression "pausa caffè" captures this idea, which refers to a coffee break that encompasses physical and cerebral rest during the day.

Another essential component of Italian cuisine is espresso. It provides the foundation for famous Italian coffee drinks like the macchiato, which is a shot of espresso "stained" with a dash of foamy milk, and the cappuccino, which is a popular breakfast drink made with equal parts espresso, steamed milk, and a crown of foam. These variants highlight how Italian espresso can be tailored to suit a wide range of palates while upholding the fundamental values of excellence and artistry.

The fact that espresso machines are so standard in Italian homes only highlights the importance of espresso in Italian society.

Italians have welcomed the ease of use and instant gratification of espresso machines for their daily fix, in contrast to many other countries where making coffee at home may require complex techniques. It is evidence of how good coffee has become more accessible, with the quest for the ideal espresso shot becoming a regular habit ingrained in family life instead of being limited to café settings.

Even though the Italian espresso culture is subject to constant change, it adapts to the changing tastes in coffee. The core of espresso culture persists even as specialty coffee and unconventional brewing techniques find their place in the Italian landscape. It symbolizes the eternal love affair between Italy and its favorite beverage and a cultural anchor that unites generations through custom and ritual.

To sum up, Italian espresso culture celebrates skill, camaraderie, and the ability to appreciate the small things in life. Every sound, from the grind of coffee to the hiss of the espresso machine to the laughter exchanged over a cup, is a part of this ageless and rich symphony. A small cup of liquid history contains unsaid poetry and all the tastes and complexity of life. To experience Italian espresso is to immerse oneself in a cultural legacy that extends beyond coffee.

## Turkish Coffee

Turkish coffee is a deeply rooted beverage with a complex preparation procedure refined over the ages, making it a revered icon in the mosaic of worldwide coffee cultures. Turkish coffee is a monument to the skill of slow brewing and the joy of community and discussion. It is as aromatic as it is ritualistic. Exploring the world of Turkish coffee reveals not only a brewing technique but also a generation-spanning cultural phenomenon.

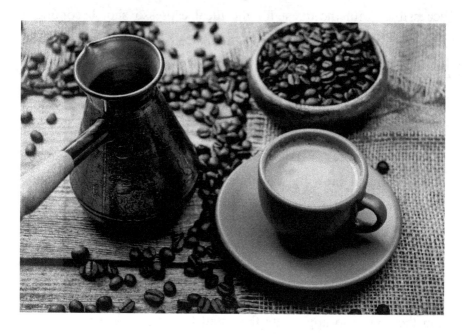

Turkish coffee is primarily made with finely ground coffee, frequently combined with cardamom to add even more taste and scent. Coffee is more than a beverage; it's a tool for forming friendships, exchanging stories, and creating the illusion of time stopping. Making Turkish coffee is a deeply traditional and valued activity that is as much a social occasion as a culinary one.

Turkish coffee combines finely ground coffee beans, usually from a dark roast, with cold water and optional sugar in a cezve, a specific kettle. This little copper or brass kettle with a long handle is necessary for the Turkish coffee ceremony. The coffee is then allowed to infuse the water and give it a rich, foamy texture by gradually bringing the liquid to a boil over low heat. The brewer must be sensitive to the minute variations in the coffee's consistency; the procedure is precise and demands patience and attention to detail.

In Turkish coffee preparation, the coffee grind is critical. The coffee is pounded to an excellent powder—almost talcum-like—so that the water may fully dissolve the coffee. Turkish coffee is known for its rich flavor and velvety texture, enhanced by this fine grind. The right coffee beans are also important; many people choose Arabica varietals because of their complex flavors.

Turkish coffee's sweetness can be adjusted, giving it a unique flavor. The amount of sweetness is specified when placing an order: sade (unsweetened), az şekerli (little sugar), orta (medium sugar), or şekerli (sweet). Sugar is added during the brewing process. This adaptability to different taste preferences reflects Turkish coffee's elasticity, making it a truly individualized experience.

The way Turkish coffee is presented is one of its distinctive features. The coffee is served in small cups known as fincans and sometimes served with a slightly sweet treat, such as Turkish delight, and a glass of water. Tassography is a unique form of fortune-telling made possible by the coffee grounds settling at the bottom of the cup. The Turkish coffee experience is made more mysterious by the belief that the coffee grounds' patterns after consumption hold glimpses of the future.

Turkish coffee is closely associated with cultural traditions, even beyond its production. Turkish coffee is traditionally made and served socially to show hospitality and promote relationships. Offering a cup of coffee is a friendly and welcoming gesture in Turkish homes, and declining one is regarded as rude. Making and serving Turkish coffee is a chance to take a moment to unwind, have deep conversations, and create enduring memories.

A place on UNESCO's Representative List of the Intangible Cultural Heritage of Humanity attests to Turkish coffee's impact on the world coffee scene. This designation recognizes Turkish coffee's cultural relevance and social traditions and its distinctive preparation process. It is evidence of the enduring appeal of this historic beverage that people worldwide still find captivating.

Traditional coffee shops, called Kahane, have functioned as gathering places for people to socialize, hold intellectual conversations, and even engage in political debate in the busy streets of Istanbul and beyond. These places, with their elaborate décor and full of people absorbed in conversation and coffee, perfectly capture the ageless appeal of Turkish coffee as a spark for neighborhood interaction.

Turkish coffee is rich and velvety; when we sip it, we become part of a centuries-old tradition. It's a ritual that helps us to be mindful of the here and now, to savor the tastes that are gradually developing on our palates, and to enjoy one other's presence. Time seems to move at a different speed in Turkish coffee—a leisurely rhythm that inspires us to stop, think, and appreciate life's richness one cup at a time.

## Latin American Coffee Traditions

With its varied and lively coffee culture, Latin America is tucked away between the tropics. The region has been a mainstay in the global coffee industry, producing some of the most renowned beans in the world, from the foggy mountains of Colombia to the sun-kissed farms of Brazil. Beyond the coffee beans, Latin American coffee customs convey a tale of affluent ancestry, deeply ingrained traditions, and an intense love for the craft of coffee that goes well beyond the cup.

Colombia is widely recognized as the birthplace of the Arabica coffee bean, and for good reason. The Andes Mountains, home to high-altitude coffee fields that yield beans with a distinctive flavor characteristic, define the Colombian coffee landscape. Beyond simple farming, Colombian coffee has become a symbol of the country's culture. Everyday life revolves around coffee, from making a "Tinto" (black coffee) in the morning to the get-togethers with friends and family sparked by a mutual love of the beverage. The Juan Valdez sign, which stands for Colombian coffee, has gained international recognition and has come to symbolize the pride and skill of Colombian coffee farmers.

Traveling north, Mexico adds its distinct touch to the coffee mosaic of Latin America. Mexican coffee has a complex flavor affected by the country's varied terrain. It is frequently grown in the shadow of beautiful woods. Native American customs and coffee growing are entwined in areas like Chiapas and Oaxaca. A classic Mexican coffee made with cinnamon and piloncillo (raw sugar), known as "Café de Olla," reflects pre-Hispanic and colonial influences. It is more than just a drink; each sip is a flavor of history and a cultural legacy.

As we move south, the world's largest coffee market is dominated by Brazil. The massive estates that crisscross Brazil form the foundation of the country's coffee traditions. Brazil's "cafezinho," a tiny, robust cup of coffee, is a daily necessity. Numerous types of coffee can be produced in the nation due to its varied terrain and temperature. Brazilian coffee culture also permeates the country's pioneering natural and pulped natural processing techniques, credited with creating the distinctive flavors that set Brazilian coffee apart.

Coffee growing in Costa Rica's highlands is not simply a business—it is a dedication to excellence. Costa Rican coffee traditions focus on developing some of the best Arabica beans in the world through careful farming methods. The "honey process," which involves leaving some mucilage from the coffee cherry on the bean while it dries, gives Costa Rican coffee a unique sweetness. Here, coffee is not just a commodity but also a source of pride for the country, with Costa Rican coffee serving as a symbol of quality and sustainability.

The small Central American nation of El Salvador has made a name for itself in the coffee industry with beans with rich flavor and sparkling acidity. The turbulent history of El Salvador is reflected in its coffee customs, which have been crucial to the nation's economic growth. Because of the volcanic soil, the typical "tall coffee" trees—a cross of Bourbon and Typica varieties—grow well and add to the distinctive terroir of Salvadoran coffee.

Guatemala's volcanic terrain has come to be associated with Antigua coffee, renowned for its bright acidity and robust body. Beyond the cup, Guatemalan coffee is experienced in the customary "cucurucho" processions held during Holy Week. In these processions, people decorate cones with vibrant fruits and candies, illustrating the mixed cultures represented in Guatemalan coffee.

Honduras, another critical figure in the Central American coffee scene, has become a significant exporter of coffee. Honduran coffee customs strongly emphasize environmentally friendly farming methods, with many producers adopting organic and shade-grown practices. The end product is a cup of coffee that honors environmental preservation while showcasing the Honduran terroir.

Frequently eclipsed by its Central American competitors, Nicaraguan coffee boasts a unique story. Although the nation's political turmoil has influenced the country's coffee customs, Nicaraguan coffee growers' tenacity is evident. After overcoming hardship, Nicaraguan beans are becoming more well-known for their distinct flavor profile, frequently highlighted by a sharp acidity and subtle chocolate overtones.

The journey of coffee in Latin America goes beyond its agriculture to include the social and communal aspects of coffee consumption.

After a meal, the customary "sobremesa," or the extended period spent at the table, is a treasured time for jokes, anecdotes, and coffee. Coffee becomes a bridge that unites people to enjoy life's little and significant milestones. It becomes a catalyst for connections.

The "cooperativa" paradigm demonstrates how coffee and community relate to Latin American coffee customs. Many small-scale coffee growers become members of cooperatives, combining resources and knowledge to overcome industry obstacles. This collaborative attitude shows a dedication to sustainability and group success, guaranteeing that the profits from the coffee trade get to the people who grow the beans.

We taste the tradition, history, and passion of the people who produce each cup of coffee as we enjoy the distinctive flavors of Latin American coffee. Turning a bean into a cup is evidence of the mutually beneficial interaction between the environment, the populace, and the cherished customs that turn coffee from a beverage into an artistic medium. In addition to enjoying coffee, Latin American coffee customs encourage us to fully engage in a cultural experience that unites people from different backgrounds, transcends national boundaries, and honors the enduring appeal of this beloved beverage.

# Chapter XII

## DIY Coffee Blends

### Blending Techniques

A harmonic and well-balanced cup of coffee is created through the skillful art of blending, which is highly regarded in the complex world of coffee production. This centuries-old custom involves more than just combining various coffee beans; it's a labor-intensive procedure that requires talent, skill, and a thorough knowledge of each bean's unique qualities. In preparing coffee, blending techniques are used to create a distinctive and memorable experience for the discriminating coffee enthusiast and achieve the ideal taste profile.

The choice of premium coffee beans is the cornerstone of a good mix. Each bean adds unique notes of body, aroma, and acidity to the blend, giving it a unique personality. Blending requires a deep understanding of the many flavors of various coffee origins. It allows the roaster to create a combination of more than the sum of its parts. The possibilities for crafting a taste masterpiece are as endless as the coffee-growing regions themselves, whether it's the earthy undertones of Indonesian types, the bright and lemony tones of Ethiopian beans, or the chocolatey richness of beans from Central America.

Combining beans with different qualities is a primary blending method to establish balance. For example, a blend may have high-acid beans to add brightness and fuller-bodied beans to balance the flavors and add depth and richness. The interaction of these contrasting components produces a well-rounded cup that appeals to the taste on several levels. The tricky part is striking that delicate balance where no flavor overpowers the others, and every element contributes to the symphony.

On the other hand, other mixes concentrate on balancing comparable flavor characteristics to highlight a specific attribute. This strategy frequently combines beans from the same area or those processed similarly. The end product is a combination that highlights a particular flavor note, such as the nutty overtones of almonds, the floral scent of jasmine, or the fruity sweetness of berries. Roasters can develop blends that highlight the best flavors within a given spectrum by choosing beans that have similar characteristics.

Roast profiles are considered during the blending process, which goes beyond the skill of taste balancing. Every coffee bean responds to roasting differently, and getting the right flavor requires an awareness of these behaviors. Darker roasts can add smokiness and caramelization, while lighter roasts may maintain the natural characteristics of the beans. Blenders work within this range to bring out or tame particular qualities, enhancing the flavor of the mix.

Blended coffees are often compared to single-origin coffees, prized for their uniqueness and purity. Blending, however, is a way to create a fresh and vibrant flavor experience rather than straying from the essence of individual beans. When carefully prepared, blends can provide complexity, depth, and a fusion of many flavor notes, enhancing the experience of drinking coffee.

The examination of processing methods is also encompassed by blending procedures. Blenders use the distinct qualities that beans with natural or washed processing impart by adding layers of complexity to the finished product. For example, a mix could have the crisp and clean qualities of soaked beans and the fruity and wine-like overtones of organically processed beans. Combining these several processing techniques adds to the blend's complexity and allure.

Demand for distinctive and creative blends is rising in today's coffee market, where specialty coffee shops and artisanal roasters are thriving. Blenders are pushing the envelope of custom, trying novel taste combinations, and exposing customers to a world of flavors they have never encountered. Due to this innovative attitude, seasonal blends, limited editions, and even partnerships between roasters and coffee producers have emerged, demonstrating the dynamic and constantly changing character of the blending craft.

Blending has made its way into the homes of coffee lovers and is no longer only the domain of professional roasters. With DIY blending, people may customize their coffee experience to suit their tastes by experimenting with different ratios and combinations to find the ideal blend. Due to their increased involvement in actively exploring flavors, consumers, and coffee have developed a stronger bond due to the democratization of blending.

Mastering blending takes time, effort, and a commitment to lifelong study, just like any other art form. Roasters and coffee lovers strive for perfection, honing their methods and learning more about coffee beans and their intricate interactions. The finest blends are not made in a vacuum but result from a roaster's close relationship with the raw material, knowledge of the roasting process, and enthusiasm for producing a coffee experience that transcends the ordinary.

To conclude, mixing coffee beans is an exquisite experience that delves into the essence of flavor and creates a harmonious blend unparalleled in taste. Blending is an art form that honors the variety of coffee, involving meticulous bean selection, thoughtful analysis of roast profiles, brilliant processing techniques, and a constant search for equilibrium. Blending is a dynamic and developing process that continues to influence the landscape of coffee culture, whether expert roasters or inquisitive home fans do it. Blending provides a canvas for taste discovery and a passport to a world of rich and complex coffee experiences.

## Creating Personalized Coffee Blends

The search for the ideal cup of coffee in the dynamic world of coffee appreciation goes beyond brewing methods and into the world of customized blends. Creating a personalized coffee blend is similar to being a skilled chef combining different ingredients to produce a flavor symphony that appeals to specific tastes. Coffee lovers may now transcend the limitations of store-bought blends and explore a world where every cup is a unique expression of flavor and personality thanks to the craft of flavor alchemy.

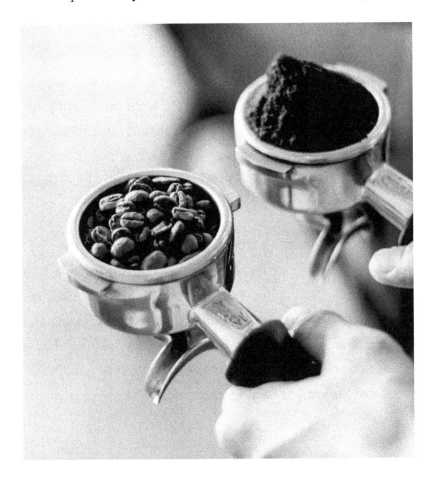

The knowledge that various coffee beans bring unique qualities to the table is the foundation of customized coffee blending. A coffee blender considers each bean's origin, roast character, and flavor notes, just like a chef chooses ingredients for a dish. Because of their unique terroirs and growing environments, single-origin beans provide a foundation for further investigation. Each type adds a layer of complexity to the blend, whether it's the earthy undertones of Sumatran coffee, the rich chocolatey notes of Colombian beans, or the fruity notes of Ethiopian Yirgacheffe.

The process of blending a custom blend starts with the coffee beans that are chosen. In-depth details regarding the flavor profiles of their beans are frequently supplied by roasters and suppliers, providing insightful information about the scents and tasting notes. Equipped with this understanding, the blender transforms into a curator, carefully selecting beans that enhance and balance one another. A harmonious and balanced marriage that is more than the sum of its parts is the aim.

The degree of roasting is a critical factor in determining the blend's flavor character. Light roasting frequently keeps the subtle flavors of the beans intact, bringing out their inherent qualities. Dark roasts provide a robust and bold taste, while medium roasts balance flavor development and bean origin. Understanding the interplay between various roast levels—a rich, caramelized depth from dark roasts or a symphony of bright acidity from light roasts—is the art of blending.

Effective coffee blending is characterized by exact measurement. To get the right balance, the amounts of each bean in the mix must be precisely measured. Careful measurement guarantees flavor consistency, enabling the blender to repeat the blend. The purposeful process of blending requires patience and an acute palate; this is where the craft of blending differs from the casual act of mixing beans.

Blending is more than just putting beans together; it's about telling a story in a cup. Every sip tells a different tale, influenced by factors including the beans' origins, the altitude at which they were cultivated, and the processing techniques used. Combining the stories of various beans, the mixer takes on the role of a storyteller and creates a sensory experience beyond the ordinary.

Creating a customized coffee blend involves more than just roasting and measuring; it also requires imagination. A coffee blender selects beans to evoke a specific sensory palette like an artist selects colors to produce a masterpiece. It's important to experiment, as this inspires blenders to push limits and find novel flavor combinations. Every iteration of this voyage of self-discovery adds fresh perspectives and perfects the mixture to suit personal tastes.

The option to customize the coffee to specific tastes is what makes making customized blends so appealing. The possibilities are as varied as the coffee landscape itself, whether one is in the mood for a dark and velvety after-dinner cup or a bright and zesty morning brew. Blenders might play around with different bean counts and ratios to satisfy their caffeine addiction until they discover a blend that suits their tastes.

Sharing a customized blend with someone special signifies intimacy among coffee connoisseurs. A well-balanced mix is more than just a drink; it's a manifestation of the passion and personality of the blender. It starts a dialogue and invites others to enjoy a well-chosen taste adventure. Personalized coffee blends encourage a sense of community by bringing people together through a mutual appreciation of the brewing craft.

Beyond the satisfaction of drinking a beautifully made cup, customizing blends fosters a closer relationship with the whole coffee-making process. It enables an awareness of the complex journey beans travel from the farm to the roastery by inviting people to explore the world of coffee from seed to cup. This newfound knowledge elevates the coffee experience by elevating each cup to celebrate skill and devotion.

Crafting bespoke blends is a testament to the endless possibilities in the world of coffee, as the demand for distinctive and individualized coffee experiences keeps rising. It's a journey that gives people the confidence to step outside of pre-packaged blends and accept coffee's alchemical role in their daily routine. The next time you have a cup of coffee, think about the creativity that goes into it—the deliberate bean selection, the exact roasting technique, and the inventive spirit that turns an ordinary beverage into a customized work of art.

# Chapter XIII

## Troubleshooting Common Coffee Issues

### Bitter Coffee

When done right, bitterness is a note that adds variety and depth to the symphony of tastes in the vast and fragrant world of coffee. But when it takes center stage and overwhelms the delicate flavors of the brew, it may make an enjoyable experience harsh. Any coffee lover who wants to become an expert brewer must comprehend the causes of bitterness in coffee, the elements that lead to its prominence, and the art of expertly balancing it.

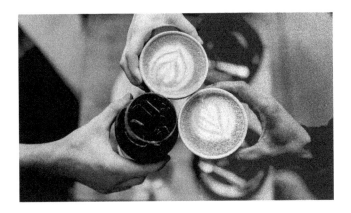

Coffee's bitterness stems from chemicals that are extracted during the brewing process. Caffeine, an alkaloid that occurs naturally in coffee beans, is one of the culprits. Although caffeine adds to the energizing properties of coffee, over-extraction during brewing can result in a strong aftertaste that lingers in the mouth. It takes careful calibration of the brewing variables to achieve that exact balance where the energizing qualities of caffeine are present but not overpoweringly bitter.

The rate at which soluble chemicals are released during the extraction process is significantly influenced by the grind size of the coffee beans. Because finely ground coffee has more surface area, extraction times can be shortened. But this also raises the possibility of over-extraction because water seeps through the ground more quickly, removing unpleasant components in addition to pleasant flavors. However, under-extraction from coarsely ground coffee might leave it tasting sour. Therefore, one of the most critical steps in reducing bitterness is finding the ideal balance by varying the grind size.

Another critical component in the bitterness equation is the temperature of the water. If it gets too hot, more bitter chemicals are extracted as the extraction process quickens. Insufficient liquid will be removed if the temperature is too low, resulting in a bland and unimpressive cup. Water temperatures between 195 and 205 degrees Fahrenheit are the sweet spot for coffee brewing. Staying within this range reduces the possibility of an excessively bitter result while allowing for the extraction of desired flavors.

Bitterness and brewing time are closely related concepts. An extended contact period between water and coffee grinds might enhance the extraction of certain chemicals, such as those that give the coffee its bitter flavor. Setting the brewing duration becomes a delicate skill in techniques where the brewer controls the water flow, such as pour-over or drip brewing. In contrast, if the grind size or pressure is not precisely adjusted when making espresso, bitterness may still come through despite the short and well-regulated extraction durations.

The bitterness profile is also greatly influenced by the coffee bean type. The beans' origin, roast level, and quality affect the flavor. Although darker roasts are well-liked for their robust and intense flavor, they frequently have a more noticeable bitterness. Conversely, lighter roasts may have more vibrant acidity and flowery overtones, reducing the prominence of anger. A discriminating coffee lover can discover the ideal balance by experimenting with various coffee varietals and roasting intensities.

The goal of addressing bitterness in coffee is to achieve a harmonious balance with other flavors rather than just trying to keep it out of the cup. The acidity, sweetness, and bitterness combination gives coffee a complex flavor profile. A trace of bitterness can be a complimentary feature that some coffee connoisseurs actively seek out, adding to the overall complexity of the cup. Each note in this interplay of flavors contributes to the overall symphony, much like the layers in a masterfully produced piece of music.

Methods like blending provide a calculated way to control resentment. A brewer can produce a synergy that lessens the prominence of any one taste by blending beans with distinct flavor profiles. The blending process opens up a world of possibilities, enabling the production of distinctive, well-balanced coffee blends that satisfy a range of palates.

A route to a softer cup is offered by alternate brewing techniques for individuals who find bitterness overpowering. For instance, cold brew produces a smoother, less bitter extraction by steeping coarsely ground coffee in cold water for a long time. Additionally, immersion methods like the French press offer another flavor profile by letting the coffee grounds rest in water before separating them.

The geography of the human palate is complex and subjective; what one person finds bitter may be the intensity that another seeks. Because of the wide range of tastes, the world of coffee is incredibly fascinating. It is not about eliminating harshness from coffee; instead, it is about negotiating its complexities to create a cup that suits individual tastes.

To sum up, coffee bitterness is a complex product of the brewing process that needs to be carefully considered and expertly manipulated. Every factor affects the delicate balance between bitterness and the other taste components, including the type of beans used, the grind's size, the water's temperature, and the brewing process's length. Accepting bitterness as a complementary element in the coffee symphony enables connoisseurs to enjoy the range of flavors this cherished beverage offers fully. Allow us to appreciate the bitter moments that enhance our coffee experience and transform each cup into a distinct and unforgettable composition as we continue to study the subtleties of brewing.

## Weak Coffee

Few things are more depressing in coffee's vast and complex world than taking that first sip of what you hoped would be a strong and stimulating brew, only to be let down by a poor cup. Coffee's weakness is not just a question of taste; it frequently indicates an imbalance in the brewing process, wherein the beverage's potential for a full-bodied, rich flavor still needs to be realized. This essay aims to solve the enigma surrounding poor coffee by examining the elements that lead to its bland taste and providing advice on turning a weak cup of coffee into an intense and fulfilling experience.

To comprehend weak coffee, one must delve into the principles of coffee extraction. Coffee brewing is fundamentally a complex dance between water and coffee grinds, whereby the soluble components in the beans are extracted to produce the beloved beverage. Under-extraction, which occurs when insufficient amounts of the coffee's solids and tastes are removed during brewing, is sometimes associated with weak coffee. Numerous factors, including the water temperature, brewing time, and coffee bean grind size, might cause this.

The grind size is one of the most critical factors in coffee extraction. Overly coarsely ground beans might lead to under-extraction, leaving the coffee weak and lacking in flavor.

Conversely, an excellent grind may result in an excessive extraction, adding bitterness to the drink. A thorough grasp of the brewing process is necessary to get the optimal grind size; for example, a coarser grind might work well in a French press, but a finer grind is better for espresso. One of the most critical steps in conquering the obstacle of weak coffee is to change the grind size to pursue a robust cup.

The proportion of coffee to water is equally significant in the quest for audacity. A weak and bland flavor can be produced by diluting the brew with too much water or coffee. On the other hand, using too many coffee grinds compared to water can result in an overwhelming bitter flavor. Finding the perfect ratio calls for accuracy and trial and error, considering it may change based on brewing technique and individual preferences.

The water's temperature is a subtle but essential element in the coffee-brewing symphony. Cold water might help extract flavors, making the coffee taste solid and exciting. Conversely, overheated water runs the risk of over-extraction, revealing harsh undertones that overwhelm the coffee's natural subtleties. The ideal water temperature between 195 and 205 degrees Fahrenheit is essential for making a more robust, more delicious cup of coffee.

The brewing time is another factor that might make the difference between weak and robust coffee. An extended brew may result in over-extraction, while a short medicine may lead to under-extraction. It takes an acute eye and an understanding of the nuances of the brewing process to perfect the delicate balance between the amount of time that water and coffee grinds are in contact. A customized technique can be achieved by experimenting with brewing times, which allows the coffee enthusiast to perfect the method and get the correct strength.

One aspect frequently overlooked in pursuing more robust coffee is the selection of coffee beans. Selecting beans that match the intended strength can have a significant influence because different beans have different flavor characteristics. For those who like a more robust cup, dark roasts, renowned for their powerful and bold flavors, can be the solution. Furthermore, experimenting with single-origin beans and mixes can enhance the flavor experience by adding more complexity to the brew.

The freshness of the coffee beans is a crucial factor in influencing the strength of the final cup, even aside from the technical requirements of brewing. Stale beans may need help to produce the robust tastes characteristic of a premium brew since they have lost their volatile chemicals and aromatic oils. A straightforward but frequently disregarded method for boosting coffee's flavor and intensity is to ensure you always have a supply of fresh coffee beans in an airtight, refrigerated container.

If you want a more robust cup, consider the brewing method you use carefully. Flavors may be extracted in various ways, and experimenting with different procedures can help you find your favorite. If you're unhappy with the intensity of your drip coffee, trying out a French press, AeroPress, or pour-over could help you get the right amount of boldness.

Weak coffee is an invitation to experiment and improve the brewing method rather than a judgment. It's a blank canvas waiting for the meticulous, adventurous, and passionate brushstrokes to turn it into a flavorful masterpiece. Accepting the shift from timid to courageous necessitates being open to learning, growing, and appreciating the finer points of the coffee-making art.

To sum up, weak coffee is a mystery that begs to be solved, and the key is to carefully balance a number of variables during the brewing process. Every component, including water temperature, brewing duration, coffee-to-water ratio, grind size, and bean selection, adds to the harmonious combination of flavors. In addition to being a technical challenge, the search for boldness in coffee is also a sensual adventure that invites connoisseurs to explore the full potential of their preferred beans and experience the fullness of a well-brewed cup.

## Other Common Problems and Solutions

Coffee lovers frequently encounter difficulties in their quest for the ideal cup, which can throw off the peaceful brewing ritual. Whether you're a novice homebrewer or a seasoned barista, obstacles will inevitably arise when producing coffee. To ensure that every cup lives up to the high expectations established by the discriminating coffee enthusiast, it is imperative to comprehend and resolve these typical issues.

A common complaint among coffee lovers is the bitterness that can ruin the otherwise enjoyable taste of a newly made cup. Over-extraction, in which unwanted compounds are extracted from the coffee grinds during brewing, is a common cause of bitterness in coffee. This might happen if you grind your coffee too finely or leave it to brew for too long. You can achieve the right balance by shortening the brewing time or increasing the grind size to counteract this. This will result in a firm but not overly bitter cup.

In contrast, one of the most frequent grievances voiced by coffee enthusiasts is the lack of flavor or intensity in their brews. Under-extraction, which occurs when the brewing process cannot extract sufficient soluble components from the coffee grinds, is often associated with this problem. It could be brought on by an excessively coarse grind size or insufficient brewing time. To fix this, try experimenting with a finer grind or brewing for a little bit longer to improve the extraction and produce a fuller and more fulfilling cup.

The problem of uneven flavor from one brew to the next is one of the subtler problems that coffee lovers deal with. Variations in water temperature, coffee-to-water ratio, and grind size can all lead to inconsistency. Carefully considering these factors is necessary to produce a consistently great cup. Achieving a consistent flavor profile in every brew requires using a dependable scale for accurate readings, keeping the water temperature steady, and grinding at the same size.

The sediment at the bottom of the cup, frequently occurring when utilizing specific brewing techniques like Turkish coffee or the French press, is a source of aggravation for coffee makers. Because these methods do not use a paper filter, some sediment is expected;

nonetheless, very gritty coffee can be unsettling. To solve this, you can enhance the overall clarity of the brew without compromising flavor by making a significant investment in a high-quality burr grinder to obtain a more uniform grind.

The unattractive sourness that occasionally taints a cup of coffee is another issue that might detract from the enjoyment of drinking coffee. Sourness is usually a sign of under-extracted or under-roasted beans during brewing. To fix this, make sure the beans are properly roasted. Try experimenting with a finer grind or longer brewing time to help balance the flavor and eliminate that unwanted harshness in your cup.

Getting the ideal foam could be difficult for those who enjoy making milk-based coffee drinks. Milk frothing irregularities can result in flat or excessively bubbly foam, which removes the velvety feel ideal for beverages like cappuccinos and lattes. The secret to perfect milk foaming is to keep the temperature at the proper level and attain the desired consistency. A rich and creamy foam that improves the whole coffee experience can be made by using fresh, cold milk and ensuring the frothing wand is clean.

Even the most seasoned coffee makers need clarification when their freshly brewed coffee smells unpleasant. This problem is usually linked to the coffee beans absorbing smells, which can happen when stored incorrectly. To avoid this, coffee beans must be kept in sealed containers away from strong-smelling materials. Furthermore, keeping the coffee maker and grinder clean regularly contributes to preserving the aroma's purity.

Problems with the equipment might be frustrating for people who like the convenience of automatic coffee makers. These issues, which might range from component malfunctions to variations in brewing temperature, can lower the quality of the brew. To guarantee constant functioning, routine maintenance is essential. Examples of this maintenance include descaling the machine and cleaning its parts. Completing the troubleshooting directions provided by the manufacturer and obtaining expert assistance when required can also aid in resolving more complicated problems.

To sum up, there are obstacles to becoming an expert coffee maker. From the overpowering bitterness that overtakes a well-meaning brew to the elusive pursuit of the ideal milk foam, a mishap offers an opportunity for improvement. Achieving the consistently great cups that every coffee fan strives to create requires understanding typical issues with coffee preparation and implementing specific remedies. Through determination, patience, and experimentation, the coffee maker can turn these difficulties into learning experiences that lead to a more satisfying and sophisticated brewing process.

# Chapter XIV

## The Sustainable Coffee Journey

### Ethical Sourcing

Ethical sourcing has come to be recognized as a critical factor influencing the coffee industry, where our senses are overwhelmed by the aroma of freshly brewed beans and the decadent richness of flavors. A global network of coffee producers, harvesters, and communities whose livelihoods are entwined with the coffee trade exists beyond the ritualistic enjoyment of a daily cup. Beyond only using high-quality beans, ethical sourcing in the coffee industry is crucial since it affects the supply chain's overall social, environmental, and economic effects.

Adherence to fair trade practices is fundamental to ethical sourcing. This calls for establishing honest relationships between buyers and producers to guarantee that coffee growers obtain a reasonable crop price. A more compassionate strategy has replaced the traditional model of taking advantage of low-income farmers, in which the profits of the coffee trade are shared more fairly among the bean growers. In addition to giving coffee growers financial security, fair trade pricing gives them the means to make community investments in sustainable farming methods, healthcare, and education.

Additionally, ethical sourcing takes into account the environmental impact of coffee production. Initiatives centered around ethical sourcing increasingly include sustainable farming practices, like organic farming and shade-grown horticulture. The primary goals are to protect soil health, conserve biodiversity, and use as little toxic fertilizers and pesticides as possible. In addition to protecting the environment, this dedication to sustainability helps produce delicious, premium beans.

Developing direct trading connections between coffee roasters and suppliers is crucial to ethical sourcing. Coffee roasters can interact directly with farmers, promoting openness and an awareness of the difficulties encountered at the source by eschewing middlemen. This close relationship guarantees that individuals who devote their time, effort, and knowledge to the bean's cultivation receive a just portion of the earnings. By working with farmers to apply best practices in planting, harvesting, and processing, roasters can also directly impact the quality of the beans.

The growth of ethical certifications like Rainforest Alliance, Fair Trade, and Organic has further demonstrated the coffee industry's dedication to ethical sourcing. Customers can be reassured by these certifications that the coffee they buy complies with social and environmental requirements. These certifications frequently include requirements for adhering to ethical labor norms, which forbid the use of child labor and guarantee safe working conditions on coffee farms, in addition to fair salaries and sustainable methods.

Beyond just taking the environment and economy into account, ethical sourcing also considers social and cultural factors. It acknowledges how crucial it is to protect the welfare and rights of the workforce in areas that produce coffee. Programs for ethical sourcing must include initiatives centered on education, community development, and gender equality. The coffee business may catalyze positive social change, strengthening communities and promoting a more equitable and inclusive coffee trade by investing in these areas.

Ethical sourcing tackles the historical injustices that have afflicted the coffee industry in addition to assisting local communities. Ethical initiatives address the colonial history of exploitation, which saw coffee-producing regions frequently subjected to unfair trading practices. Through recognition of the past and efforts to correct these disparities, the industry hopes to create a more equitable and inclusive coffee market that respects the worth and contributions of all parties.

Customers are a significant factor in the movement toward ethical sourcing. There is a greater need for coffee that comes from ethical sources as people become more conscious of the influence of their decisions. Because of this, many coffee lovers deliberately search for companies that share their beliefs and select goods with transparent sourcing information and ethical certifications. Demand for ethical coffee from consumers drives responsible behavior and motivates more coffee growers to use fair trade and sustainable practices.

However, there are obstacles to the coffee industry's mainstream adoption of ethical sourcing. A smooth transition is hampered by the complexity of international supply chains, fluctuating economic situations, and the requirement for systemic adjustments. However, the dedication to ethical sourcing is only growing due to the realization that a flourishing coffee industry is based on justice, sustainability, and shared wealth.

In summary, ethical sourcing in coffee production is a dedication to promoting a fair and sustainable coffee industry that goes beyond the act of brewing coffee. Proper pricing, environmental stewardship, social responsibility, direct trade links, and other aspects are all part of the complex strategy known as ethical sourcing, which aims to change the coffee supply chain altogether. As we enjoy our daily cup, we can support a worldwide movement that honors the richness of the lives and communities that grow this treasured bean and the richness of flavor in our coffee.

## Sustainable Practices

The coffee industry must embrace sustainability in a world with an endless need for coffee. Sustainable coffee-making methods are more than just a fad; they signify a fundamental change toward ethical and responsible production that upholds the environment, strengthens local communities, and guarantees the continued existence of the cherished coffee bean.

The idea of ethical sourcing is central to the creation of sustainable coffee. This entails growing coffee beans with an emphasis on the welfare of the farmers and the environment. Environmental deterioration and unfair business activities have occurred in the traditional coffee industry. However, the sustainable coffee movement aims to address these problems by supporting organic cultivation, fair trade, and certifications that ensure adherence to moral standards.

A key component of sustainable coffee production is organic cultivation. Using organic coffee beans instead of synthetic fertilizers and pesticides improves soil health and biodiversity. This preserves the health of both growers and customers and the natural ecosystem surrounding coffee plants. The unique flavor profile of organic coffee, which reflects its terroir, is evidence of the coexistence of agriculture and the environment.

An additional essential component of sustainable coffee practices is fair trade certification. This initiative fosters equitable economic relationships by guaranteeing that coffee farmers are fairly compensated for their efforts. Coffee growers who engage in fair trade can invest in their communities, supporting infrastructure development, healthcare, and education. The appropriate trade certification acts as a beacon, directing customers toward coffee options consistent with their values as they prioritize ethical purchases.

The trend for coffee grown in shade is an example of an environmentally responsible farming method. Large land areas are cleared for coffee plantations to cultivate coffee in a monoculture. On the other hand, the coffee produced in the shade promotes planting coffee beneath the existing tree canopies. This promotes biodiversity by protecting natural ecosystems and giving migratory birds a place to live. The slower maturing phase of the beans under the shade is responsible for the distinctive flavors found in the final coffee.

Sustainability in coffee manufacturing and transportation goes beyond the era of cultivation. The amount of water used in the manufacturing of coffee can have a significant impact on the environment. Reusing and treating water is one-way sustainable processing methods reduce the impact on nearby water supplies. Additionally, efforts like carbon-neutral shipping and roasting procedures are used to reduce carbon footprints, making sure that the environmental impact of coffee manufacturing is minimized throughout the process.

The third-wave coffee movement has been instrumental in changing the coffee business by prioritizing sustainability, traceability, and quality. This trend encourages consumers to follow the path of their coffee from farm to cup and promotes supply chain transparency. The third wave ensures that sustainability is an integral part of the story of coffee production and not just a label by encouraging direct partnerships between roasters and growers.

Reusable and compostable coffee packaging is becoming increasingly common, indicating a shift in consumer preferences toward sustainability. Customers are looking for brands that share their environmentally conscious beliefs as awareness of the adverse effects of single-use packaging on the environment rises. In addition to cutting waste, sustainable packaging shows a dedication to environmental responsibility on all fronts.

In conclusion, adopting sustainable methods for producing coffee is a step toward turning the sector into a force for good. Every stage of the coffee-making process, from the sun-dappled slopes where coffee plants flourish to the ethical decisions made by customers, works toward a day when coffee is not just a beverage but also a force for social justice and environmental preservation. One sip at a time, by embracing sustainability, we produce a cup of coffee and a dedication to a better, more just world.

## Eco-friendly Brewing Options

The coffee industry is not immune to the trend in public consciousness toward more sustainable methods. Coffee lovers are looking for environmentally friendly brewing choices that make a delicious cup of coffee and help the environment since they are becoming more conscious of their influence on the environment. Every step of the coffee-making process, from bean to cup, offers the chance to make decisions that are kind to the environment.

The first step in producing environmentally friendly coffee is choosing your beans. Choosing coffee beans that are organically certified or made using sustainable agricultural methods guarantees that the cultivation process has the minimum possible environmental damage. These beans frequently originate from farms that value biodiversity, avoid using dangerous pesticides, and use moral labor practices—a comprehensive strategy that goes beyond the simple act of brewing.

Going on to the brewing procedure, switching to reusable coffee pods instead of single-use ones is one of the most straightforward yet significant environmentally responsible decisions you can make. Single-use pods need energy-intensive processes during production, making up a sizable portion of landfill garbage. Reusable solutions significantly lessen the environmental impact of your everyday brew, such as metal filters for pour-over systems or refillable capsules. This change results in a fresher and more customized cup by reducing waste and giving more control over the coffee grinds utilized.

Besides utilizing reusable pods, selecting the proper brewing apparatus can be crucial in advocating sustainability. Purchasing coffee makers with programmable functions and low energy usage can reduce waste. In addition, manual brewing techniques like pour-over or French press don't use power, making them a greener option for individuals who like a more hands-on coffee ritual.

Another factor in environmentally friendly brewing is water usage. Water conservation and practical use are crucial factors to consider during brewing. Water waste can be reduced by employing easy techniques like pouring over ways with a kettle with a precise spout to prevent overpouring. Furthermore, recycling and reusing water from different phases of the coffee-making process for other domestic purposes is a prime example of the inventive spirit that guides sustainable brewing.

Beyond the brewing process, there's also an opportunity to make environmentally friendly decisions when disposing of coffee grounds. Used coffee grounds can be recycled into a rich fertilizer for plants or utilized for various do-it-yourself home projects instead of ending up in the trash. Coffee grinds can be recycled to close the loop and transform waste into a valuable resource.

Additionally, adopting the idea of "zero waste" in coffee preparation calls for careful packaging selection. Selecting coffee companies that value environmentally friendly and biodegradable packaging materials lessens the effect your coffee consumption has on the environment. A few businesses have also unveiled cutting-edge package designs that emphasize recycling and reduce waste.

To summarize, environmentally friendly coffee brewing choices use a holistic approach that considers the entire process from bean to brew, not just the coffee in the cup. Making sustainable decisions at every level helps significantly lessen our coffee consumption's impact on the environment. As lovers of coffee, we may appreciate the atmosphere and enjoy our favorite beverage. In addition to enjoying a good cup of coffee, we can help create a more sustainable and environmentally friendly coffee culture by adopting eco-friendly brewing techniques.

# Conclusion

Through the pages of "Coffee Making Recipes: Brewing Perfection," we've taken a trip beyond the simple process of making coffee—a journey into the worlds of sustainability, art, and culture. As we end this extensive tutorial, the secret to making the ideal cup of coffee at home is to embrace a newfound passion for the craft rather than just following recipes.

This book aims to be your companion in the search for coffee excellence, from the methodical pour-over technique, where every drop of water becomes a brushstroke in a flavor masterpiece, to the discovery of many coffee cultures worldwide. The chapters have been organized to provide information, methods, and a passion for the ideal cup of coffee, regardless of your level of experience—whether you're a beginner looking to learn the fundamentals or an expert desiring new heights in your coffee experience.

However, the story goes further than the contents of your coffee mug. We've looked into environmentally friendly coffee brewing solutions since enjoying coffee shouldn't come at the expense of the environment. We've looked at how adopting sustainable methods can make every cup a deliberate decision for a cleaner future, from choosing beans that come from ethical sources to cutting waste and energy use.

We hope that as you close the pages of this book, you will enjoy the trip as much as the finished brews—the aromatic dance of coffee beans, the healing pour-over rituals, and the delight of sharing your creations with other coffee lovers. The coffee-making industry is dynamic and constantly changing, and you may use this guide to explore flavors, methods, and cultural quirks.

May the perfume of freshly ground coffee fill your mornings, the warmth of a well-made espresso decorate your afternoons, and the inventiveness of flavored blends illuminate your evenings. Let this book begin a never-ending journey into the art of coffee making, where every cup serves as a canvas, every brew offers the chance to hone your craft, and every sip is an opportunity to relish the pure joy of a well-made beverage.

After all, the trip never ends; it just gets better with every drink. May you have infinite success in your coffee-making attempts, and may the aroma of your masterpieces fill your home with the comforting perfume of a perfectly brewed cup. This cup represents not simply a daily ritual but also a celebration of art, culture, and a long-lasting love for the bean. I toast to your unwavering quest for the ideal brew!

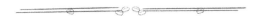

*Thank you for buying and reading/listening to our book. If you found this book useful/helpful please take a few minutes and leave a review on Amazon.com or Audible.com*
*(if you bought the audio version).*

Printed in the USA
CPSIA information can be obtained
at www.ICGtesting.com
CBHW072151280624
10819CB00016B/688